THE ANTI INFLAMMATORY COOKBOOK
COLLECTION

THE BEST RECIPES FROM
THE FAST & FRESH ANTI-INFLAMMATORY COOKBOOK &
THE ANTI-INFLAMMATORY COOKBOOK FOR TWO

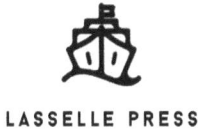

LASSELLE PRESS

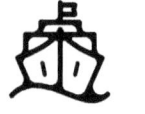

LASSELLE PRESS C<u>O</u>

© Copyright 2016 by Lasselle Press

All rights Reserved. No part of this book may be reproduced in any form without permission in writing from the author. Reviewers may quote brief passages in reviews.

Limit of Liability / Disclaimer: No part of this publication may be reproduced or transmitted in any form or by any means, mechanical or electronic, including photocopying or recording, or by any information storage and retrieval system, or transmitted by email without permission in writing from the publisher. While all attempts have been made to verify the information provided in this publication, neither the author nor the publisher assumes any responsibility for errors, omissions or contrary interpretations of the subject matter herein. The information in the book is for educational purposes only. It is not medical advice and is not intended to replace the advice or attention of health-care professionals. This book is sold with the understanding that the publisher is not engaged in providing legal, medical or other professional advice or services. Consult your physician before beginning or making any changes in your diet. Specific medical advice should be obtained from a licensed health-care practitioner. The Publisher will not assume any liability, nor be held responsible for any injury, illness or personal loss due to the utilization of any information contained herein. Adherence to all applicable laws and regulations, including international, federal, state and local laws governing professional licensing, business practices, advertising and all other aspects of doing business in the US, Canada, UK or any other jurisdiction is the sole responsibility of the purchaser or reader. Lasselle Press publishes its books in a variety of print and electronic formats. Some content that appears in electronic books may not be available in print, and vice versa.

ISBN-13: 978-1911364146
ISBN-10: 1911364146

CONTENTS

INTRODUCTION | 4

CHAPTER 1
UNDERSTANDING INFLAMMATION | 5

CHAPTER 2
BENEFITS OF THE ANTI-INFLAMMATION DIET | 11

CHAPTER 3
DIET STAPLES | 14

CHAPTER 4
ANTI-INFLAMMATION 7 DAY MEAL PLAN | 23

CHAPTER 5
BREAKFAST | 28

CHAPTER 6
BRUNCH | 50

CHAPTER 7
SOUPS & STEWS | 64

CHAPTER 8
DRINKS & SMOOTHIES | 80

CHAPTER 9
BEEF & PORK | 100

CHAPTER 10
POULTRY | 115

CHAPTER 11
SEAFOOD | 132

CHAPTER 12
VEGETARIAN | 154

CHAPTER 13
SALADS | 173

CHAPTER 14
SIDES | 188

CHAPTER 15
DESSERTS | 217

CONVERSION CHARTS | 243
BIBLIOGRAPHY | 245
INDEX | 246

INTRODUCTION

Welcome!

For many of us, inflammation can cause problems and symptoms that may be uncomfortable, painful or even unbearable. This is why we have selected the best recipes from two of our best-selling anti-inflammatory cookbooks, The Fast & Fresh Anti-Inflammatory Cookbook and The Anti - Inflammatory Cookbook For Two, here in this Collection.

We know that changing your diet and lifestyle can seem extremely daunting and so hopefully the guidance provided here in this cookbook can help make those changes easier. With this cookbook, you can continue to enjoy delicious meals with your loved one, family and friends, whilst at the same time reducing inflammation, becoming pain free and improving your overall health.

Thank you for purchasing this book and we hope that the information and recipes provided can help you get started, or continue, along the journey to improve your health and live well.

The Lasselle Press Team

I

UNDERSTANDING INFLAMMATION

This chapter will address what inflammation actually is and the problems and symptoms that can be caused by chronic inflammation, in order to help you gain a better understanding of what may be going on in your body.

WHAT IS INFLAMMATION?

Inflammation is an auto-response system used by the body to remove toxins and repair damaged tissue as a result of illness or injury. It is an essential part of the body's healing process and is usually a positive reaction.

Let's take for example your knee becoming injured - when this happens, the body's immune system works to heal the knee itself. The knee may become swollen; chemicals such as histamine, bradykinin, and prostaglandins are released as a cell is damaged and these chemicals will protect the body from further harm by causing the tissues to swell.

In turn, these chemicals are actually used to signal to the body that it needs help, and it needs help fast. The white blood cells recognize this recovery response, and attack any germs or bacteria present. The dead cells can be seen in the form of puss, which is then pushed out of the body either through coughing up phlegm, mucus, or puss.

This is usually always your body's way of protecting itself and is the natural response to injury. For many, the worst they might feel is a little bit of pain, which is called acute inflammation, and is a completely normal and healthy response.

But what if the inflammation doesn't go away?

What if the body's defence becomes its downfall?

That's when problems start. This prolonged inflammation is the type of inflammation discussed in this book. This is called chronic inflammation, and it is the symptoms and problems such as joint damage, digestive issues, cardiovascular problems and other diseases which come hand-in-hand with chronic inflammation that has most likely led you to pick up this book.

CAUSES OF CHRONIC INFLAMMATION

These range from lasting injuries, infections, toxin exposure or other autoimmune diseases.

SYMPTOMS OF ACUTE INFLAMMATION

Redness,
Pain in and around the affected area,
Increase in body temperature,
Swelling,
These symptoms are usually experienced as a result of a viral infection or injury and will usually heal in due course without intervention.

SYMPTOMS OF CHRONIC INFLAMMATION

Chronic pain around the joints,
High blood pressure,
Redness and intense heat,
Intense swelling,
Tumours in extreme cases,
Loss of function of the joint/affected area,
Food allergies,
Obesity,
Ulcers and skin problems such as dry skin, rashes, or puffy red eyes.

If you have any of these symptoms you should consult a doctor who can advise further but they may be down to chronic inflammation.

INFLAMMATION AND DISEASE

Now let's take a look into what can happen to the body over time when suffering from chronic inflammation. Examples of illnesses and diseases that have been linked to chronic inflammation are as follows:

AUTOIMMUNE DISEASES: When our body's immune system is flawed and unable to tell the difference between our own cells and foreign cells, it will attack cells in our own body using auto-antibodies. The immune system does not work as it should do as a result, and effectively works against your body. There are more than 80 known types of autoimmune disease. Normally, the common autoimmune diseases that can be caused by inflammation are multiple sclerosis, Crohn's disease, diabetes, and celiac disease. These are all autoimmune disorders that affect different parts of the body. Some of these (like celiac disease for example) are caused by food, in this case gluten, and you can help alleviate the symptoms through your dietary choices which will help lessen the inflammation.

MULTIPLE SCLEROSIS: According to the US National Library of Medicine, MS is a severe auto-immune disease affecting the brain and spinal chord and damaging the protective sheaf around nerve cells. This damage is caused by inflammation and can occur around the brain, optic nerve or spinal chord. Whilst it is not know for certain what causes MS, it has been put down to a gene or virus defect and even the environment.

DIABETES: Type 2 diabetes can be caused by a number of different factors and inflammation is one of those that can have a serious impact on diabetes because of insulin resistance in the body. Generally those with type 2 diabetes are advized to lose weight and reduce their intake of sugary and salty foods but now that studies have linked inflammation with diabetes, clearly there is good reason to choose the anti-inflammatory diet in order to improve symptoms or even prevent them.

RHEUMATOID ARTHRITIS: Causes pain and inflammation of the joints. Most people take medications for arthritis but there is a link between the disease and diet which is now recognized by many dieticians and doctors. Sometimes sugar, dairy, and processed foods are what can aggrevate or cause the inflammation, and that's why so many people are suffering needlessly when simple dietary changes could make a real difference.

ASTHMA: A chronic condition that can cause breathing problems when air passages become restricted due to inflammation. Asthma causes coughing and shortness of breath as well as attacks in those who suffer severely.

OBESITY: There has been evidence to show a direct link between chronic inflammation and obesity: inflammation can cause insulin resistance, which in turn means the body stores more fat. Furthermore, chronic inflammation can even prevent us from being able to regulate our appetites as inflammation sends signals to the brain causing resistance to Leptin (the hormone that tells your brain that you're full up). This, in turn, causes weight gain. Because of this, having too much fat, teamed with inflammation, can wreak havoc on the body.

ALLERGIES: Allergies are our body's reaction to certain proteins such as food, dust mites or pollen. When someone with an allergy is confronted with one of these proteins, allergens trigger the immune response, causing the body to go into self-defence mode. You may have experienced this in terms of sneezing, a blocked nose, and even swollen airways.

HEART DISEASE: It's the number one killer of people in the world today, and the inflammation of tissues can affect the heart, which can cause heart attacks, stroke and even heart failure; sometimes the chemicals that are released to fight the problem can build up in the cells, thus restricting blood flow and making the threat to the heart more severe.

CANCER: Research and studies have shown that 'chronic inflammation can predispose an individual to cancer'.

This doesn't even begin to account for the other problems caused by or linked to inflammation such as Alzheimer's, Parkinson's, and depression. Simply put, chronic inflammation can create horrible symptoms and even diseases, and if not controlled, can get progressively worse.

The good news is that once you understand what's causing your symptoms or illness, you can try the anti-inflammatory cookbook to eat well, reduce inflammation and in turn, improve your health.

It is always recommended to consult your doctor or dietician for advice and diagnosis before you begin, however the recipes featured in this book are all healthy, delicious and natural and therefore good for you and the rest of the family.

INFLAMMATION AND FOOD

There are many causes of inflammation including injury, sickness and strained muscles. But, if you have chronic inflammation, your allergies and reactions could also be caused by food.

You may have started to experience some of the previous symptoms when you have eaten certain foods, as there is a direct correlation between our diets and inflammation in the body. Hence the reason your diet is so important. Our bodies are designed to absorb proteins, fats, carbohydrates, vitamins, and minerals and anything we don't need is usually flushed out of the body through the digestive system. However, some toxins cause problems because they stay in the body when they shouldn't, thus triggering an immune response such as inflammation to try and get rid of these toxins, which will usually cause some kind of damage to the body.

Toxins are actually more prevalent than you might realize; there are over 100 toxins that are present within the body at any time. These toxins range from chemicals commonly found in the various pesticides sprayed on food, food dyes, specific metals that aren't supposed to be in the body, and the most common toxin of all - preservatives. Preservatives are used in many food products, even some of the whole grain and soy products that you wouldn't typically associate with toxins or chemicals. These preservatives are used to ensure a longer shelf life are are either natural (i.e. salt) or chemical. It's obviously mainly the chemical preservatives that are most harmful but excess salt can too have adverse effects on our bodies.

The body fights to get rid of these toxins and usually it is successful in doing so but with modern food and agriculture processes and an increase in packaged and ready-to-eat foods, our diets include so many toxins nowadays, that it's almost impossible for the body to eradicate them all.

Research and studies have revealed that a 'traditional Mediterranean' diet with a high ratio of monounsaturated to saturated fats and polyunsaturated fats , plenty of fruit and vegetables, legumes and wholegrains has shown 'anti-inflammatory effects when compared with typical North American and Northern European dietary patterns'. Overall your diet is key to feeling better, inside and out!

II
THE BENEFITS OF THE ANTI-INFLAMMATION DIET

In this chapter, the benefits of the anti-inflammatory diet and recipes will be covered so that you can make the choice to eat the right foods for you and start the process of reducing inflammation and the symptoms you have experienced.

BENEFITS OF THE DIET

The anti-inflammatory diet is used to help reduce the amount of inflammation in the body by removing the foods that typically cause inflammatio, thus reducing symptoms experienced and improving overall health. Benefits of the anti-inflammatory diet are revealed below:

LESSEN THE RISK OF EXPERIENCING FURTHER ILLNESS OR DISEASE

Reducing your inflammation will further help you lessen your risks of experiencing one or more of the problems aforementioned including obesity and allergies. If you're at risk of heart disease, predisposed to diabetes, have high blood pressure, or even experiencing stiff and painful joints, then this diet is for you. It will help you reduce inflammation, and you should feel significantly better over time.

LOSE OR MAINTAIN WEIGHT IN A HEALTHY WAY

Likewise, if you're trying to lose weight, you might not have considered typically inflammatory foods as being the problem, as they aren't always associated with weight-gain. Instead you may have been trying to control your calorie intake and doing more exercise, whilst struggling to lose any significant weight. Now, this isn't a fad diet and you probably won't drop a pant size in two weeks. But that's not the purpose of this change as there are many more benefits of losing weight gradually and changing your eating habits long term. The healthy foods used in this cookbook will help you lose weight and reduce inflammation.

PREVENT FOOD ALLERGIES

As previously stated, the anti-inflammatory diet can also help with food allergies. Allergies can be problematic for many people, and if they're severe enough, they can be life threatening. Reducing inflammation can help minimise the severity or regularity of allergic reactions you experience.

GREAT FOR GLUTEN FREE

For many people who have a gluten allergy, this book can also help you. A lot of the time people may not recognize gluten as a problem until they're on this diet or a gluten-free diet. The anti-inflammatory nature of this diet can actually help relieve the symptoms experienced by those who are intolerant to gluten.

IMPROVE YOUR SKIN

Alongside all of these benefits, the diet can also greatly improve skin. Sometimes, inflammation can cause dry and ageing skin and you might also have noticed redness, and even problems such as rosacea of the skin, all of which which can be caused by inflammation. This diet can help improve your skin's appearance, meaning you'll feel and look younger!

INCREASE YOUR ENERGY LEVELS

Moreover your energy will increase. Sometimes, we can feel our energy sap because of the foods that cause inflammation. It's not just sugars that sap our energy but processed foods as well. You are what you eat as the old adage goes, and sometimes eating foods that cause tiredness and fatigue can be a major issue. These foods can also make you feel depressed. However, with the inflammation diet, you can say goodbye to lethargy and depression through eating foods that give you energy and improve your quality of life.

REDUCE SYMPTOMS

Then there is the pain and soreness you may be experiencing. You shouldn't have to live with chronic pain and if you're not eating the right foods then your symptoms will certainly be worse than they need to be. Pain shouldn't take over your life, and you can make sure that it doesn't through the recommended foods and meals provided in this cookbook.

BE THE HAPPIEST AND HEALTHIEST VERSION OF YOURSELF

Making your own well-informed choices can change your life for the better. Try this diet and you will soon realize the potential that your body and mind have, and what you've been missing out on all this time. Don't let your health get in the way of feeling happy – eat well, live well and be well!

III
DIET STAPLES: WHAT TO KEEP IN YOUR KITCHEN

Now that you know about the diet and its benefits, it's important to go over what foods and ingredients you should keep in your kitchen, as well as those which are best limited or avoided all together.

FOODS TO AVOID OR CUT DOWN:

Try keeping a food diary, where you log what you have had to eat and drink each day, as well as a detailed description of your symptoms and how you feel. That way you can start to track which foods seem to work well with you and your body and which do not in order to make informed decisions as to the best foods and ingredients for you.

HYDROGENATED OILS AND TRANS FATS:

These are found in many of the baked goods that we know and love. They are one of the main causes of inflammation in the body, which can be problematic. You commonly find these in cookies, cakes and breads, and while they might taste good, they are best avoided because your body can't break them down properly.

SUGAR:

Now, not all sugars are bad but we typically consume a diet loaded in sugar. Definitely cut out synthetic sugars and try to reduce natural sugars such as honey to a minimum or a special treat!

SYNTHETIC SWEETENERS:

Sugar replacements such as aspartame, saccharin, sucralose and other chemicals found in diet sodas or sugar-free foods are toxic, and part of the reason why inflammation occurs in the first place. Avoid these chemicals like the plague if you can. Replace these with honey, maple syrup, and stevia if you need something sweet.

MEAT:

Not necessarily bad for you, but it can cause inflammation for some people. Commercial meat is what usually causes inflammation, as these animals are not typically fed on a healthy diet. If you do eat meat, go for grass-fed, hormone-free meat instead.

DAIRY:

Can cause sensitivity, especially the reactions to the casein proteins in cows' milk. If you do experience discomfort when eating dairy, then it's best if you avoid it.

MERCURY:

Can be found in fish such as swordfish, and while having a little is okay, too much can be problematic. Limit this to once a month.

GLUTEN:

Wheat can cause sensitivity in many people, and gluten can be inflammatory even for those who don't have the gluten allergy or celiac disease. Wheat is also a problem when it's been modified, as it can cause toxins to build up in the body. You should also watch out for white flour, because it breaks down quickly, spiking your blood sugar levels, causing crashes and energy slumps soon after.

NIGHTSHADES:

Fruits and vegetables are encouraged on this diet, but nightshades can be a problem for some people. These are usually eggplants, potatoes, peppers, and tomatoes. They contain alkaloids, which can cause inflammation in those susceptible to them. There is some debate on this, as many have unique anti-inflammatory properties of their own. If you are unsure, eliminate one at a time from your diet and monitor in your food log to see if this makes a difference.

OMEGA 6:

Causes high cholesterol and cardiovascular disease. The Western diet includes high levels of omega 6. Ideally, you should aim for a ratio of 1:1 between omega 3 and omega 6. You should try to avoid many of the seed and vegetable oils if you can, as these can cause a build up of omega 6 in the body.

PROCESSED FOODS:

Start to avoid these; it's not easy to do so at first because we are so reliant on them for quick and easy meals as part of a busy lifestyle. However, if you are able to avoid them, your symptoms should reduce dramatically.

ALCOHOL:

Make sure that you don't consume too much alcohol as it causes inflammation. Aim for 1-2 drinks a week i.e glass of wine/pint of beer/spirit.

FOODS TO BUY:

These are foods you should immediately add to your shopping list. Replace the banned items with these and incorporate them into your daily diet right away!

WHOLE FRESH FOODS:

You can have meat, poultry, veggies, fruits and fish. Ideally, buy all of these organic, gluten-free, and grass-fed/free-range as these are foods in their natural states, without added chemicals and sugars. If budget is an issue, stick to fresh fruit and vegetables over tinned and limit your intake of meat and poultry so that you have less but of a better quality.

FRUIT AND VEGETABLES:

These should be the staple of your diet as they include vital nutrients and help to keep you fit and healthy as well as having multiple benefits for skin, hair, and increased energy levels. Particularly choose:

TOMATOES: Rich in Vitamin C and cancer fighting but be careful as these are one of the nightshade vegetables. Keep a track of your foods in a food diary to see what works for you. You can eat these raw or cooked.

LEAFY GREENS: Choose spinach and collards as their high Vitamin E content has been said to protect the body from the cells that cause inflammation. The calcium levels will also help supplement your diet if you do decide to go dairy free.

STRAWBERRIES, RASPBERRIES AND BLUEBERRIES: Looking out for the vibrant colors of fruits and vegetables is often a sign of their goodness.

GARLIC AND ONIONS: Both work at shutting down the process leading to inflammation.

BEETS: High in antioxidants and anti-inflammatory, beets also help protect against heart disease and cancer.

MUSHROOMS: With so many varieties, mushrooms have anti-inflammatory properties and are an exciting and almost meaty addition to your meals. Great if you decide to cut out animal products completely.

WHOLE GRAINS: Choose unrefined wholegrains such as oatmeal and quinoa (avoid white breads and flours). These should have no added sugars on the label.

BEANS AND LEGUMES: You should eat these as part of a balanced diet because they're high fiber content which will help detox the waste out of your body. These should be eaten in moderation – stick to 1 serving per day.

HEALTHY FATS:

Not all fat is bad. You shouldto include good fats, such as omega-3 fatty acids and unsaturated fats in your diet. Some of the fatty foods to choose a few times a week are:

HEALTHY FATTY FISHES HIGH IN OMEGA 3: SALMON, MACKEREL, TUNA, SARDINES – these should be eaten 2-3 times per week in order for the anti-inflammatory properties to do their magic! Fish oil supplements can also be taken on a low meat and fish diet and have beneficial effects, especially for rheumatoid arthritis sufferers.

OLIVE OIL/COCONUT OIL: Choose one or both of these as your main oils. Coconut oil is one of the healthiest fats out there and can be used for dressings, shallow frying and as part of your beauty regime!

ALMONDS AND WALNUTS: These nuts have a whole host of benefits including high antioxidant levels. Other nuts are also anti-inflammatory.

HERBS AND SPICES:

Use herbs and spices such as cloves, ginger, cumin, turmeric and rosemary (all of which are listed as the top 4 anti-inflammatory spices following a study by The University of Florida et al).

LOW-FAT DAIRY:

If keeping dairy in your diet, it is advised that you opt for low-fat or non-fat milk and yogurt option.

UNPROCESSED SOY PRODUCTS:

These are particularly beneficial for women in reducing inflammation because of the isoflavens (which are similar to the female hormone estrogen). Choose from soy milk, edamame beans and tofu. Also great if you're going vegetarian.

YOU SHOULD START TO THROW AWAY FOODS THAT AREN'T ON THE GOOD LIST OR PERHAPS DONATE THEM TO A LOCAL HOMELESS SHELTER OR FRIEND.

KEEP ANY OF THE GOOD FOODS THAT YOU HAVE ON THE LIST AND USE THIS AS A SHOPPING LIST FOR YOUR NEXT TRIP TO THE STORE OR MARKET.

COOKING METHODS:

So what are the best cooking methods when preparing anti-inflammatory meals?

WHEN COOKING, TRY TO LIMIT THE AMOUNT OF FRYING YOU DO AND IF FRYING IS NECESSARY, USE OLIVE OIL OR COCONUT OIL.

A lot of the unhealthy fat can linger on food and nutrients are also decreased when frying. Baking, steaming or boiling are better methods for cooking with steaming being the best way to preserve vitamins and nutrients in fruit and vegetables as well as the healthiest way of cooking meats and poultry.

LIMIT THE AMOUNT OF SALT AND SUGAR YOU ADD TO FOODS WHEN COOKING, IF YOU USE THEM AT ALL.

Spices can be used to flavor your foods in place of these and are healthy to consume on the anti-inflammatory diet. Obviously if you know you're allergic to any spices in particular, please avoid these in your own cooking.

10 TIPS FOR THE ANTI-INFLAMMATION DIET:

I   HAVE AT LEAST 25 GRAMS OF FIBER EACH DAY

This is one of the most important tips as a high fiber diet will help with reducing inflammation. You should eat plenty of whole grains, fruits and vegetables as your fiber sources.

II   HAVE AT LEAST NINE SERVINGS OF FRUITS AND VEGETABLES EACH DAY.

You're probably wondering why we focus so much on fruit and veg in this diet. It's simple: they're anti-inflammatory foods and high in antioxidants. One serving = 1/2 cup of cooked vegetables or cup of raw vegetables. Add spices to liven up the taste and increase antioxidant levels.

III   HAVE AT LEAST FOUR SERVINGS OF BOTH ALLIUMS AND CRUCIFERS EACH WEEK.

Now, you're probably wondering what both of these are. Alliums are garlic, leeks, scallions and onions. Crucifers are vegetables such as cabbage, mustard greens, cauliflower, broccoli, and brussel sprouts. These all lower your risk of cancer, and help with inflammation. If you have four servings of these per week, the powerful antioxidants will be better able to elimate toxins from your body.

IV   LIMIT SATURATED FAT TO 10% OF YOUR DIET.

Only have red meat once a week and make sure to mix it with herbs, spices, and even unsweetened fruit juice to help with the toxic compounds that are released when cooking.

V OMEGA 3 FATTY ACIDS ARE YOUR FRIEND!

If you are wondering what type of fat you should have, look no further than omega 3 fatty acids. This is the type of fat you should be consuming and for good reason too. If you have a large amount of omega-3 fatty acids, you will reduce inflammation in many different areas and it can help with many chronic diseases. Choose flax meal, beans of any kind, and walnuts as well as certain fish along with an omega 3 or fish oil supplement.

VI EAT FISH AT LEAST THREE TIMES EACH WEEK

As previously explored, fish contains a host of nutrients, is generally low in calories in comparison to other meats, and is an unsaturated 'good' fat. Oily fish as well as cold-water fish are great additions to the diet.

VII CHOOSE THE RIGHT OILS

Fat is used to help with metabolic processes, and your cells need it to survive. Ideally choose olive oil and coconut oil and buy organic where you can.

VIII DON'T BE AFRAID TO SNACK

You can have a snack twice a day on this diet, and you should aim to have snacks that are healthy and include food types on the good food list. In many cases, you should go for fruit, plain Greek yogurt, or raw fruit and vegetables and nuts.

IX   AVOID PROCESSED FOODS

Processed foods and refined sugars are a big no-no on this diet. Foods that have high in fructose or sodium will also cause the chronic inflammation to spike. You should try to avoid refined sugars when you can, and you should start to read the labels on the products that you already have. Get rid of artificial sweeteners altogether.

X   CUT OUT TRANSFATS

In 2006, the FDA demanded that food companies identify transfats on their nutrition labels. The protein in transfats called a C –reactive protein can cause inflammation in the body. Not to mention, transfats open the door to a lot of other diseases such as heart disease and diabetes. You should get into the habit of reading the labels on the foods you eat and checking for "hydrogenated" or partially hydrogenated oils". These should be avoided for instance in shortenings, some margarines, cookies, and crackers.

I hope these tips help with getting started to stock up your kitchen and cook healthy meals that you can continue to enjoy alone and with those around you, whilst being safe in the knowledge that you are eating the right foods to reduce your symptoms and become pain free.

The following chapter will provide you with a 10 Day Meal Plan and Shopping List to get you ready to go!

IV
THE ANTI-INFLAMMATORY DIET
7-DAY MEAL PLAN

IN SUMMARY:

- Your food choices are key to your health and can help reduce inflammation and thus the symptoms it causes.

- Along with a healthy diet and correct treatment, reducing inflammation can help prevent diseases and illnesses such as obesity and heart disease.

- Always choose whole, natural and unprocessed foods.

- Eat a diet high in fiber.

- Choose healthy unsaturated fats over saturated fats.

- Use herbs and spices to season instead of salt and sugar.

- Eat an array of colorful fruits and vegetables.

- Vary your diet so that you are including a combination of vitamins and nutrients needed to stay healthy.

- This is not a 'weight-loss' diet but is healthy and manageable and you will feel great for it and most likley lose any unwanted pounds in the process .

- The diet will help to 'flush out' the unwanted toxins in your body.

- Keep yourself hydrated and aim to drink at least 8 glasses of water each day.

- Choose green tea, sparkling water, fruit-infused water such as water with lemon or lime, and some very diluted juices, such as pomegranate or cherry juice.

- Drink coffee sparingly and try to avoid alcohol and sodas.

- Choose supplements such as a multivitamin. If you don't eat a lot of oily fish, you should take a fish oil supplement too.

LIFESTYLE:

Exercise is important and keeps you fit and healthy. It is important you don't over-stress your body however, as this can lead to inflammation. Walking, light jogs and exercise routines such as yoga and pilates are less strenuous but just as rewarding options. Consult your doctor for further guidance on this subject.

Avoid smoking and drinking too much alcohol. These things may seem rewarding and fun in the moment but the effects they have on your body and overall healthare just not worth it.

7-DAY MEAL PLAN

This meal plan is simple to follow, and the dishes aren't too hard to make.

WEEKLY MENU

Monday

Drink before Breakfast: Glass of water with Lemon

BREAKFAST: Coconut Breakfast Burst.

LUNCH: Shrimp and Zucchini Noodle Jar.

DINNER: Nut Crusted Tilapia And Kale

Tuesday

Drink before breakfast: Glass of water with some lemon

BREAKFAST: Zucchini & Sweet Potato Frittata

LUNCH: Spiced Ginger and Carrot Soup

DINNER: Baked Garlic Halibut

Wednesday

Pre-Breakfast food: Glass of water with lemon

BREAKFAST: Tasty Gluten-Free Crepes

LUNCH: Tasty Thai Broth

DINNER: Med -Veg Lasagna

Thursday

Pre-Breakfast drink: Glass of water with lemon

BREAKFAST: Blueberry Brain Booster

LUNCH: Burrito Bowl

DINER: Sundried Tomato and Nut Pasta

Friday

Pre-breakfast drink: Glass of lemon water or lime water

BREAKFAST: Perfect Fruit Punch Pancakes

LUNCH: Shitake Squash Soup

DINNER: Italian Chicken Zucchini Spaghetti

Saturday

Pre-Breakfast: Glass of water with lemon

BREAKFAST: Blueberry & Spinach Shake

LUNCH: Vegetarian Tagine

DINNER: Pan Seared Salmon on Baby Arugula

Sunday

Pre-breakfast: Glass of water with lemon

BREAKFAST: Avocado Boats

LUNCH: A salad of kippers with celery

DINNER: Spanish Shrimp

Snacks

Feel free to have pick between 1 - 2 snacks per day between meals - See the Sides & Snacks chapter for ideas!

BREAKFAST

TROPICAL COCONUT DELIGHT

SERVES 2   PREP TIME: 2 MINUTES   COOK TIME: 10 MINUTES

A tropical fruity twist on your usual boring breakfast porridge.

- 2 CUPS WHOLEMEAL OATS
- 1 TBSP MILLED CHIA SEEDS
- 3 CUPS COCONUT MILK
- 3 TSP RAW CACAO (OPTIONAL)
- 1/2 TSP STEVIA
- 1 TSP COCONUT SHAVINGS
- 6 FRESH CHERRIES

In a pan mix the oats, cacao, stevia and coconut milk.

Heat on a medium heat and then simmer until the oats are fully cooked through (5-10 minutes).

Pour into your favorite breakfast bowl and sprinkle the coconut shavings, cherries, and milled chia seeds on top.

If you've got a sweet tooth or fancy an extra treat, try adding cacao or a drizzle of honey to serve.

WARMING GINGERBREAD OATMEAL

SERVES 2   PREP TIME: 2 MINUTES   COOK TIME: 8 MINUTES

A winter warmer – delicious for breakfast or a supper-time treat by the fire!

- 3 CUPS WATER OR SOY MILK
- 2 CUPS STEEL CUT OR WHOLEMEAL OATS
- 1 TBSP GROUND CINNAMON
- 1 TSP GROUND CLOVES
- 1/4 TSP GINGER (FRESH AND GRATED)
- 1/4 TSP GROUND ALLSPICE
- 1/4 TSP NUTMEG
- 1/4 TSP CARDAMOM
- 1 TSP HONEY TO TASTE

Mix the oats and water in a saucepan and gently heat on a medium heat for 5-8 minutes or until cooked through.

Whilst cooking stir in the spices.

When cooked and hot through, pour into your bowl.

Drizzle honey over the top if desired.

MINI FRUIT MUFFINS

SERVES 2   PREP TIME: 10 MINUTES   COOK TIME: 20 MINUTES

This is a tasty gluten and dairy-free muffin recipe - perfect for anti-inflammation.

- 1 CUP ALMOND MEAL
- 3 TSP STEVIA
- 2 TBSP CHOPPED CRYSTALIZED GINGER
- 1 TBSP GROUND LINSEED MEAL
- 1/2 CUP BUCKWHEAT FLOUR
- 1/4 CUP BROWN RICE FLOUR
- 2 TBSP ORGANIC CORN FLOUR
- 2 TSP GLUTEN-FREE BAKING POWDER
- 1/2 TSP GROUND CINNAMON
- 1 CUP SLICED RHUBARB
- 1 APPLE, PEELED AND DICED
- 1/3 CUP ALMOND MILK
- 1/4 CUP EXTRA VIRGIN OLIVE OIL
- 1 FREE RANGE EGG
- 1 TSP VANILLA EXTRACT

Preheat oven to 350°f/180°c/Gas Mark 4. Line muffin tins with coconut or olive oil using a baking brush or kitchen towel. Put the almond meal, stevia, ginger, and the linseed into a bowl.

Sieve the flours over the mix along with the baking powder and spices – stir. Add the rhubarb and the apple into the flour mixture.

In a separate bowl, beat the egg, vanilla, milk, and oil until combined. Fold the wet ingredients into the dry ingredients until smooth.

Pour batter into the muffin tin, leaving a 1 cm gap at the top so that the muffin can rise and then bake for 20 minutes or until risen and golden. Remove and place on a cooling rack before serving.

HANDY TIP: You can use a combination of any gluten free flours you can get your hands on as substitutes to the ones on this list.

BRILLIANT BUCKWHEAT BREAKFAST

SERVES 2   PREP TIME: 10 MINUTES   COOK TIME: 45 MINUTES

This is a fun and tasty granola dish that is perfect for breakfast

1 CUP WHOLEMEAL OR STEEL CUT OATS	1/3 CUP CHOPPED STRAWBERRIES OR RASPBERRIES
1/3 CUP BUCKWHEAT	1/2 CUP OF PEELED AND FINELY CHOPPED APPLES
2 CUPS WATER	
1/3 CUP SUNFLOWER SEEDS	5 TBSP COCONUT OIL
1/3 CUP PUMPKIN SEEDS	4 TBSP CACAO POWDER
	1 TSP GINGER (FRESH AND GRATED)

Preheat the oven to 350°f/180°c/Gas Mark 4.

Meanwhile mix the oats, buckwheat, and seeds into a bowl.

Put the berries, apples, coconut oil and water in a pan, cover and simmer for 10-15 minutes on a medium-high heat until the fruits are soft to touch. Then stir in the ginger.

Add the fruit mixture to a blender with the cacao and blend until smooth. Mix the fruits with the buckwheat.

Grease a baking tray with coconut oil and then spread the granola mixture on top using a knife or spatula to create a thin layer. Bake for 45 minutes.

Stir the mixture every 15 minutes so it doesn't burn. When crispy all over, remove the tray and allow to cool.

NUTMEG & CHERRY BREAKFAST QUINOA

SERVES 2   PREP TIME: 2 MINUTES   COOK TIME: 20 MINUTES

A complete protein, quinoa tastes brilliant sweet and savory and provides you with the energy you need. The cherries are a brilliant anti-inflammatory food.

- 1/2 CUP QUINOA
- 1/2 CUP UNSWEETENED FRESH CHERRIES
- 1 CUP WATER
- 1/4 TSP GROUND NUTMEG
- 1/2 TSP VANILLA EXTRACT

Get a pan and combine all of the ingredients, cooking over medium to high heat until boiling.

Once boiling, cover and simmer for 15 minutes or until the quinoa is soft and the liquid has been absorbed.

Pour into serving bowls and enjoy.

FRESH & LEAN SAUSAGE BREAKFAST

SERVES 4   PREP TIME: 8 MINUTES   COOK TIME: 15 - 20 MINUTES

Sausages are usually processed and should be avoided to fight inflammation but this recipe allows you to carry on indulging in your favorite foods.

- 2 CUPS OF LEAN GROUND PORK
- 2 TSP FRESH CHOPPED SAGE LEAVES
- 1 TSP CHOPPED THYME
- 1 TSP GROUND BLACK PEPPER
- 1/4 TSP GROUND NUTMEG
- 1/4 TSP CAYENNE PEPPER
- 1/4 TSP CHOPPED ROSEMARY
- 1 TBSP EXTRA VIRGIN OLIVE OIL

Get a mixing bowl and add all of the ingredients.

Mix with a spoon or blender until blended and form 8 patties using the palms of your hands to shape.

Heat the oil in a skillet, over a medium heat and cook the patties for 9 minutes one side and 9 on the other side until they're browned and cooked through.

GLUTEN-FREE VANILLA CREPES

SERVES 2   PREP TIME: 5 MINUTES   COOK TIME: 10 MINUTES

These tasty crepes are great for anyone who is on the anti-inflammation diet or not. Delicious and healthy!

- 2 FREE RANGE EGGS
- 1 TSP VANILLA
- 1/2 CUP NUT MILK OF YOUR CHOICE
- 1/2 CUP WATER
- 1 TSP MAPLE SYRUP
- 1 CUP GLUTEN-FREE ALL-PURPOSE FLOUR
- 3 TBSP COCONUT OIL

In a medium bowl add the eggs, vanilla, nut milk, water, and syrup together until combined. Add the flour to the mix and whisk to combine to a smooth paste.

Take 2 tbsp of the coconut oil and melt in a pan over a medium heat.

Add 1/2 crepe mixture and tilt and swirl the pan to form a round crepe shape.

Cook for about 2 minutes until the bottom is light brown and comes away from the pan with the spatula.

Flip it and cook for a further 2 minutes.

Serve and repeat with the rest of the mixture!

MEDITTERANEAN VEGETABLE FRITTATA

SERVES 2   PREP TIME: 10 MINUTES   COOK TIME: 30 MINUTES

A zesty veggie treat, great on its own for breakfast or as a side with your favorite meal.

- 1 TBSP COCONUT OR EXTRA VIRGIN OLIVE OIL
- 4 FREE RANGE EGGS
- 1 SWEET POTATO, PEELED AND SLICED USING POTATO SLICER OR SHARP KNIFE.
- 1 PEELED AND SLICED ZUCCHINI
- 2 TSP PARSLEY
- 1 TSP CRACKED BLACK PEPPER

Preheat broiler on a medium heat.

Heat the oil in a skillet under the broiler until hot.

Spread the potato slices across the skillet and cooking for 8-10 minutes or until soft.

Add the zucchini to the skillet and cook for a further 5 minutes.

Meanwhile, whisk the eggs and parsley in a separate bowl, and season to taste before pouring mixture over the veggies in the skillet.

Cook for 10 minutes on a low heat until golden.

Remove and turn over onto a plate or serving board.

AVOCADO BOAT BREAKFAST

SERVES 2   PREP TIME: 2 MINUTES   COOK TIME: 4 MINUTES

Poach the egg and float it in its own avocado boat; full of healthy fats and protein to start your day. Remember to have an egg only once or twice a week.

---

1 RIPE AVOCADO

2 FREE RANGE EGGS

1 TBSP WHITE WINE VINEGAR

Place a large pan of water on a high heat and boil.

Once boiling add white wine vinegar (don't worry if you don't have it, it just helps with the poaching).

Lower the heat to a simmer and crack the eggs in. Top tip: do it quickly and from a height to get a nice round shape.

Stir the water ever now and then around the eggs to keep them moving and cook for 2 minutes for a very runny yolk; 2-4 minutes for a soft to firm yolk and 5 for a hard yolk.

Whilst cooking, prepare your avocado by cutting through to the stone lengthways around the whole of the fruit.

Use your palms on each side to twist the avocado and it should come away into 2 halves. Using your knife, carefully wedge it into the stone and pull to remove the stone. Alternatively, cut around the stone with the knife and use the sharp end to coax it out.

Use your avocado halves as a dish for the eggs and serve.

CITRUS YOGURT BIRCHER

SERVES 2   PREP TIME: 2 MINS (REST OVERNIGHT IF POSSIBLE)   COOK TIME: NA

This is a tasty fruity breakfast salad, high in antioxidants.

---

1 CUP OF STEEL CUT OATS

1 PINK GRAPEFRUIT PEELED AND SLICED (IF YOU CAN'T GET GRAPEFRUIT TRY MANGO OR LEMONS)

2 ORANGES PEELED AND SLICED

16 OZ. LOW FAT GREEK YOGURT

HANDFUL OF FRESH CRANBERRIES OR CHERRIES FOR TOPPING

Mix the oats and fruit with the yogurt and allow to soak for as long as possible (overnight is best).

Serve and top with honey and cranberries or cherries if desired – the oats should be nice and mushy and will have soaked up the flavors of the fruit.

APRICOT & VANILLA PANCAKES

SERVES 2   PREP TIME: 4 MINUTES   COOK TIME: 4 MINUTES

You don't have to stop eating your favorite sweet breakfasts on an anti-inflammatory diet; try making these and you'll be surprised. This mixture serves around 4 pancakes

---

- 1/3 CUP BUCKWHEAT, BANANA OR ALMOND MEAL FLOUR
- 1 FREE RANGE EGGS
- 1/2 CUP ALMOND, HAZELNUT OR SOYA MILK
- 1/2 TSP GLUTEN FREE BAKING POWDER
- 1 APRICOT PEELED AND CUBED
- 1 PEACH PEELED AND CUBED
- 1 TSP VANILLA EXTRACT
- 1 TBSP LOW FAT GREEK YOGURT TO SERVE
- 1 TSP COCONUT OIL

Preheat oven on low.

Whisk all the ingredients (apart from the greek yogurt) until light and fluffy.

Leave to one side (you don't need to leave over night, they'll be just as scrummy!)

Heat coconut oil in a pan over a medium heat.

Pour 1/4 of the mixture into a pancake shape and cook for 30 seconds to a minute.

Flip and repeat.

Stack on a plate and keep warm in an oven on a low heat.

Repeat until you've used rest of the mixture.

Serve with a dollop of greek yogurt and extra fruit if wished.

You can make extra and keep in a sealed container in the fridge for 2-3 days.

CHIA BERRY SUPERFOOD

SERVES 2   PREP TIME: 2 MINS   COOK TIME: NA

This is a healthy and filling breakfast food that's so simple to make.

---

1 LARGE GREEN OR RED APPLE, PEELED AND SLICED	2 CUPS FRESH ORGANIC BLUEBERRIES
1 TBSP CACAO POWDER	1/2 CUP ALMONDS, RAW AND CHOPPED
10 PITTED RAISINS	2 TBSP CHIA SEEDS
10 RASPBERRIES	

Add half the blueberries and apples to a sealed container.

Separately, add the rest of the blueberries with raisins and raspberries and blend until smooth.

Add the blended mix to the apple and blueberries and pour in the chia seeds.

Serve the mix and top with the crushed almonds and a dusting of cacao powder.

This can be kept in a sealed container in the fridge for up to 2-3 days.

MARVELLOUS MINI MEATLOAVES

SERVES 2 PREP TIME: 10 MINUTES COOK TIME: 30 MINUTES

Scrumptious, meaty treats.

- 1/2 CUP LEAN GROUND TURKEY
- 1/2 CUP SKINLESS GROUND CHICKEN
- 1/4 CUP COCONUT MILK
- 1 MINCED GARLIC CLOVE
- 1/4 CUP CHIVES, FINELY CHOPPED
- 1 TBSP PAPRIKA
- SPRINKLE OF CHOPPED PARSLEY
- SPRINKLE OF BLACK PEPPER
- 1 TSP COCONUT OIL

Preheat the oven to 400°f/200°c/Gas Mark 6.

Mix turkey, chicken, garlic, chives, paprika, and coconut milk together, mixing until the ingredients hold.

Season with black pepper to taste.

Line a muffin tin with coconut oil and divide the mixture into each hole.

Bake in the oven for 30 minutes or until the meat is cooked through.

Sprinkle cooked meatloaves with parsley and serve alone or with side salad.

SWEETCORN & MUSHROOM FRITTATA

SERVES 4   PREP TIME: 5 MINUTES   COOK TIME: 30 MINUTES

A healthy snack great for any time of the day!

- 1 TBSP COCONUT OIL
- 1/2 CUP SWEETCORN (FRESH FROM THE COB OR FROZEN)
- 10 DICED MUSHROOMS
- 6 EGGS
- 1 CUP COCONUT MILK
- SPRINKLE OF PEPPER
- 2 CUPS ARUGULA

Preheat the broiler to a medium heat.

Whisk the eggs and coconut milk in a separate bowl.

On a medium heat, heat the coconut oil in an oven proof (steel) frying pan, adding in the sweet corn and the mushrooms, and sautéing for 5 minutes.

Add the egg mix to the pan and cook on a low heat for 7 minutes until it becomes light and bubbly.

Finish the frittata in its pan under the broiler for a further 5 minutes or until crispy on the top and cooked right through.

Serve with a side or arugula

PROTEIN SCOTCH EGGS

SERVES 2   PREP TIME: 10 MINUTES   COOK TIME: 25 MINUTES

These tasty protein breakfast foods are great for those on the go and won't flare up your symptoms.

- 16 OZ LEAN GROUND TURKEY
- 1/2 TSP BLACK PEPPER
- 1/2 TSP NUTMEG
- 1/2 TSP CINNAMON
- 1/2 TSP CLOVES
- 1/2 TSP DRIED TARRAGON
- 1/2 CUP FRESH PARSLEY, FINELY CHOPPED
- 1/2 TBSP DRIED CHIVES
- 1 CLOVE GARLIC, FINELY CHOPPED
- 4 FREE RANGE EGGS, BOILED AND PEELED

Preheat the oven to 375°F/190°C/Gas Mark 5.

Cover a baking sheet with parchment paper.

Combine the turkey with the cinnamon, nutmeg, pepper, cloves, tarragon, chives, parsley and garlic in a mixing bowl and mix with your hands until thoroughly mixed.

Divide the mixture into 4 circular shapes with the palms of your hands.

Flatten each one into a pancake shape using the backs of your hands or a rolling pin.

Wrap the meat pancake around 1 egg, until it's covered. (You can moisten the meat with water first to help prevent it from sticking to your hands).

Bake in the oven for 25 minutes or until brown and crisp – check the meat is cooked through with a knife before serving.

PINEAPPLE & CHIA OATS

SERVES 2   PREP TIME: 2 MINUTES   COOK TIME: 10 MINUTES

A wholesome fruity breakfast!

- 2 CUPS WHOLEMEAL (GLUTEN-FREE) OATS
- 1 TBSP MILLED CHIA SEEDS
- 3 CUPS COCONUT MILK
- 3 TSP RAW CACAO (OPTIONAL)
- 1/2 TSP STEVIA
- 1 TSP COCONUT SHAVINGS
- 1/2 CUP PINEAPPLE

In a pan mix the oats, cacao, stevia and coconut milk.

Heat on a medium heat and then simmer until the oats are fully cooked through (5-10 minutes).

Pour into your favorite breakfast bowl and sprinkle the coconut shavings, pineapple, and milled chia seeds on top.

If you've got a sweet tooth or fancy an extra treat, try adding cacao to serve.

GINGER & BLUEBERRY MUFFINS

SERVES 2 PREP TIME: 10 MINUTES COOK TIME: 20 MINUTES

Gorgeous breakfast muffins.

- 1 CUP ALMOND MEAL
- 3 TSP STEVIA
- 2 TBSP CHOPPED CRYSTALLIZED GINGER
- 1 TBSP GROUND LINSEED MEAL
- 1/2 CUP BUCKWHEAT FLOUR
- 1/4 CUP BROWN RICE FLOUR
- 2 TBSP ORGANIC CORN FLOUR
- 2 TSP GLUTEN-FREE BAKING POWDER

- 1 CUP BLUEBERRIES
- 1/3 CUP ALMOND MILK
- 1/4 CUP EXTRA VIRGIN OLIVE OIL
- 1 FREE RANGE EGG
- 1 TSP VANILLA EXTRACT

Preheat oven to 350°f/180°c/Gas Mark 4. Line muffin tins with coconut or olive oil using a baking brush or kitchen towel. Put the almond meal, stevia, ginger, and the linseed into a bowl.

Sieve the flours over the mix along with the baking powder and spices – stir. Add the rhubarb and the apple into the flour mixture.

In a separate bowl, beat the egg, vanilla, milk, and oil until combined. Fold the wet ingredients into the dry ingredients until smooth.

Pour batter into the muffin tin, leaving a 1 cm gap at the top so that the muffin can rise and then bake for 20 minutes or until risen and golden. Remove and place on a cooling rack before serving.

HANDY TIP: You can use a combination of any gluten free flours you can get your hands on as substitutes to the ones on this list.

SESAME SEED & CHERRY OATS

SERVES 2   PREP TIME: 10 MINUTES   COOK TIME: 45 MINUTES

Fruity buckwheat breakfast.

---

1 CUP WHOLEMEAL GLUTEN FREE OATS

1/3 CUP BUCKWHEAT

2 CUPS WATER

1/3 CUP SESAME SEEDS

1/3 CUP PUMPKIN SEEDS

1/2 CUP OF CHERRIES

5 TBSP COCONUT OIL

Preheat the oven to 350°f/180°c/Gas Mark 4.

Meanwhile mix the oats, buckwheat, and seeds into a bowl.

Put the berries, apples, coconut oil and water in a pan, cover and simmer for 10-15 minutes on a medium-high heat until the fruits are soft to touch. Then stir in the ginger.

Add the fruit mixture to a blender with the cacao and blend until smooth. Mix the fruits with the buckwheat.

Grease a baking tray with coconut oil and then spread the granola mixture on top using a knife or spatula to create a thin layer. Bake for 45 minutes.

Stir the mixture every 15 minutes so it doesn't burn. When crispy all over, remove the tray and allow to cool.

Serve as a crispy breakfast treat alongside low fat yogurt and fresh fruit if desired.

TASTY BANANA CREPES

SERVES 2   PREP TIME: 5 MINUTES   COOK TIME: 10 MINUTES

Gluten free treats.

- 2 FREE RANGE EGGS
- 1 TSP VANILLA
- 1/2 CUP NUT MILK OF YOUR CHOICE
- 1/2 CUP WATER
- 1 TSP MAPLE SYRUP
- 1 CUP GLUTEN-FREE ALL-PURPOSE FLOUR
- 3 TBSP COCONUT OIL
- 1 BANANA, SLICED

In a food processor blend the eggs, vanilla, nut milk, banana and water until combined.

Add the flour to the mix and combine to a smooth paste.

Take 2 tbsp of the coconut oil and melt in a pan over a medium heat.

Add 1/2 crepe mixture and tilt and swirl the pan to form a round crepe shape. Cook for about 2 minutes until the bottom is light brown and comes away from the pan with the spatula.

Flip it and cook for a further 2 minutes.

Repeat with the rest of the mixture and serve with maple syrup (optional).

PERFECT PEACH PORRIDGE

SERVES 2   PREP TIME: 5 MINUTES   COOK TIME: 20 MINUTES

Nutritious and filling buckwheat porridge.

- 1/2 CUP BUCKWHEAT
- 1/2 CUP PEACHES, SLICED
- 1 TBSP MAPLE SYRUP
- 1 1/2 CUPS ALMOND MILK
- 2 CUPS WATER

Bring the water to a boil on the stove, add the buckwheat and place the lid on the pan.

Lower heat slightly and allow to simmer for 7-10 minutes, checking to ensure water does not dry out.

When most of the water is absorbed, remove from the heat and allow to sit for 5 minutes.

Drain any excess water from the pan and stir in the almond milk, heating through for a further 5 minutes.

Now add the peaches and maple syrup.

Serve warm!

MIGHTY EGGS & SPINACH

SERVES 2   PREP TIME: 10 MINUTES   COOK TIME: 25 MINUTES

Prepare these in advance for a quick breakfast or mid morning snack.

- 16 OZ LEAN GROUND TURKEY
- 1/2 TSP BLACK PEPPER
- 1/2 TSP NUTMEG
- 1/2 TSP CINNAMON
- 1/2 TSP CLOVES
- 1/2 TSP DRIED TARRAGON
- 1/2 CUP FRESH PARSLEY, FINELY CHOPPED
- 1/2 TBSP DRIED CHIVES
- 1 CLOVE GARLIC, FINELY CHOPPED
- 4 FREE RANGE EGGS, BOILED AND PEELED
- 1/2 CUP SPINACH

Preheat the oven to 375°F/190°C/Gas Mark 5.

Cover a baking sheet with parchment paper.

Combine the turkey with the cinnamon, nutmeg, pepper, cloves, tarragon, chives, parsley and garlic in a mixing bowl and mix with your hands until thoroughly mixed.

Divide the mixture into 4 circular shapes with the palms of your hands.

Flatten each one into a pancake shape using the backs of your hands or a rolling pin.

Wrap the meat pancake around 1 egg, until it's covered. (You can moisten the meat with water first to help prevent it from sticking to your hands).

Bake in the oven for 25 minutes or until brown and crisp – check the meat is cooked through with a knife before serving.

Wash the spinach and serve eggs on a bed of spinach.

BRUNCH

MIDDLE EASTERN CHICKEN SALAD

SERVES 2   PREP TIME: 10 MINUTES   COOK TIME: 10-15 MINUTES

Asian inspired chicken salad.

- 2 BONELESS, SKINLESS CHICKEN BREAST HALVES
- 1 TBSP OF CILANTRO, FRESHLY CHOPPED
- 2 TBSP. FRESHLY SQUEEZED LEMON JUICE

FOR THE MARINADE:
- 1/2 CUP LOW FAT GREEK YOGURT
- 1 TBSP TURMERIC
- 1/4 TSP CUMIN
- 1/2 TSP GINGER, GRATED
- 1/2 TSP PAPRIKA
- SPRINKLE OF GROUND PEPPER
- 1 TSP EXTRA VIRGIN OLIVE OIL
- 1/4 CUP WATER

FOR THE SALAD:
- 1/2 CUCUMBER, DICED
- 1 CUP WATERCRESS OR RAW SPINACH
- 1/2 CHOPPED ONION

Add the spices to the yogurt in a mixing bowl before adding the chicken and covering.

If time allows, marinate for one hour up to overnight but don't worry if you need to cook right away!

Preheat broiler to a medium heat and grease a baking tray with olive oil. Shake off the excess marinade from the chicken and then grill for 10 minutes (turning once half way). Check the meat is cooked and piping hot in the middle before removing from broiler and placing to one side.

Carefully slice chicken.

Meanwhile layer the salad onto serving plates and squeeze over the juice of your lemon.

Add afresh finely chopped cilantro to serve.

CHINESE SPICED SALMON

SERVES 2   PREP TIME: 10 MINUTES   COOK TIME: 40 MINUTES

A fresh oriental staple with mustard - a superhero in the anti-inflammatory world.

- 2 SWEET POTATOES
- 1 TSP HOT PREPARED CHINESE MUSTARD
- 1/2 CUP CHINESE BROCCOLI OR RAPINI
- 1 TSP YELLOW MUSTARD SEEDS
- 2 5 OZ. ALASKAN SALMON FILLETS

Preheat the oven to 400°f/200°c/Gas Mark 6.

Wrap the sweet potatoes in foil and roast in the oven for about 40 minutes or until tender.

Meanwhile, grind the mustard seeds in a pestle and mortar or blender and then rub over the salmon fillets.

Place the salmon fillets into the oven (wrapped in parchment paper for extra moisture) and cook for 12-15 minutes or until cooked through.

Meanwhile, boil a pan of water on a high heat and steam the broccoli over for 8-10 minutes or until tender before setting aside.

Remove sweet potatoes once cooked and allow to cool before scooping out the flesh and pureeing in a blender until smooth.

Stir in the mustard with the sweet potato puree.

Serve the salmon fillets on a bed of broccoli and sweet potato puree on the side.

CURRIED CHICKPEAS AND YOGURT DIP

SERVES 2   PREP TIME: 10 MINUTES   COOK TIME: 15 MINUTES

Vegetarian and deliciously moreish – packed full of protein and anti-inflammatory spices.

- 1/2 ONION, PEELED AND CHOPPED
- 1 TSP GARLIC, PEELED AND MINCED
- 2 TBSP COCONUT OIL
- 1 TBSP CURRY POWDER
- 1 TSP CUMIN
- 1/2 TSP TURMERIC
- 1/4 TSP CAYENNE PEPPER
- 2 BEEF TOMATOES, CHOPPED
- 1 TBSP CILANTRO

- 1 CAN OF CHICKPEAS (DRIED IF YOU WISH BUT REMEMBER TO SOAK OVERNIGHT!)
- 1/2 CUP LOW FAT GREEK YOGURT
- 1/2 CUCUMBER, DICED
- 1 SPRIG OF FRESH MINT, RIPPED INTO SMALL PIECES WITH YOUR FINGERS
- 1/2 FRESH LEMON

For the salad:

Heat the oil in a skillet over a medium-low heat. Sweat the onion and garlic for 3-4 minutes, stirring until softened.

Add the curry powder and cumin to the onions and cook for about 2 minutes, whilst stirring as you smell the beautiful release of flavors!

Add in the tomatoes and cook over a medium high heat, stirring until the mix has thickened. Add the chickpeas to the tomato mix before adding in the rest of the cilantro and spices and cooking for 5-6 minutes before covering and simmering on a low heat while you prepare the dressing.

For the dressing:
Meanwhile prepare the topping by stirring together the yogurt, cucumber, mint, and juice of ½ lemon. Serve the chickpeas warm with a dollop of the dressing.

SIRACHA STEAK WRAPS

SERVES 2   PREP TIME: 10 MINUTES   COOK TIME: 25 MINUTES

This is a filling and healthy wrap.

---

1 1/2 CUPS OF LEAN BEEF, CUT INTO STRIPS

1 LARGE WHITE ONION, DICED

1 CLOVES OF GARLIC, DICED

2 TBSP SIRACHA

2 TSP SESAME OIL

HANDFUL OF PEA SHOOTS OR CRESS

4 LARGE ICEBERG, ROMAINE, OR LETTUCE LEAVES FOR THE WRAPS

Heat 1 tsp oil in a pan on a high heat, and then add the beef and cook for 12-15 minutes.

In a separate pan, heat 1 tsp oil and add the onions, cooking on a medium heat until browned for about 5 minutes. Add the onions to your beef.

Now add in the garlic, sesame oil and siracha to the mix and stir.

Remove from the heat and layer your ingredients inside the lettuce leaf.

Sprinkle over the pea shoots/cress before wrapping the lettuce around the beef like you would a fajita.

Serve your lettuce wraps warm and enjoy with your hands!

SHRIMP AND ZUCCHINI NOODLE JARS

SERVES 2   PREP TIME: 5 MINUTES   COOK TIME: 20 MINUTES

These shrimp noodles are fantastic in a jar and can be transported to work easily – say goodbye to your soggy sandwiches!

- 3 CLOVES OF GARLIC, CRUSHED
- 1 TBSP COCONUT OIL
- 12 JUMBO SHRIMPS
- 1 ONION, FINELY SLICED
- 1 ZUCCHINI, SPIRALIZED OR CUT INTO THIN STRIPS
- 1 CARROT, SPIRALIZED OR CUT INTO THIN STRIPS
- 1/2 LIME

(FOR THE SEASONING)
- 1 TSP PAPRIKA
- 1/2 TSP CAYENNE PEPPER
- DASH OF CHILLI FLAKES

Combine the ingredients for the seasoning in a bowl and then add the shrimp and coat.

Heat the coconut oil and garlic in a pan on a medium to high heat, and then add the onion, sautéing for 2 minutes.

Add the dressed shrimp and cook until opaque.

Add the zucchini noodles for 3 minutes and saute.

Add to a sealable glass jar and layer carrot slices on top with the juice of your lime.

SPANISH LANGOUSTINE PAELLA

SERVES 2   PREP TIME: 15 MINUTES   COOK TIME: 40 MINUTES

A Mediterranean Masterpiece! Peppers can be taken out if you find they flare up your symptoms. They have been noted for their anti-inflammatory vitamins, but like any other food, need to be monitored.

- 2 TBSP EXTRA VIRGIN OLIVE OIL
- A HANDFUL OF BLACK OLIVES
- 1 ZUCCHINI CUT INTO CUBES (ABOUT HALF CM THICK)
- 2 BELL PEPPERS CUT INTO CUBES (ABOUT HALF CM THICK)
- 1 TBSP PAPRIKA
- 3 LARGE ORGANIC TOMATOES CUT INTO EIGHT PIECES
- 6OZ LANGOUSTINES - BUTTERFLIED
- 1 FRESH LEMON, CUT INTO QUARTERS
- A HANDFUL OF COOKED FRESH PEAS

Heat oven to 325°f/170°c/Gas Mark 3. Oil a baking tray and add the tomatoes, pepper, olives and zucchini.

Drizzle a little more olive oil over vegetables and sprinkle paprika over the top.

Oven bake for 30-40 minutes.

Whilst your vegetable mix is roasting, butterfly your langoustines: pull off the head and legs with your fingers and leave the tails on for presentation.

Score down the centre of each langoustine (do not slice in half) and then pull open on each side of the score to flatten.

Turn the oven up to 350°f/180°c/Gas Mark 4 and add to a roasting tray with an extra drizzle of olive oil. Cook for 10 minutes, ensuring prawns are piping hot before serving.

Serve the roasted vegetables (with added peas) in a pasta/rice dish with the prawns on top and the lemon chunks for squeezing. Add salt and pepper to taste.

ORIENTAL CABBAGE & EGG ROLL

SERVES 2   PREP TIME: 5 MINUTES   COOK TIME: 15 MINUTES

Protein packed and tasty.

- 1 HEAD OF CABBAGE, CUT INTO SLICES
- 1 CARROT, CUT INTO SLICES
- 1 TBSP COCONUT OIL
- 1 TBSP SESAME OIL
- 4 GREEN ONIONS, DICED
- 2 LARGE FREE RANGE EGGS

Boil a pan of water on a medium high heat and add the eggs.

Cook for 5 minutes for a runny yolk or 7 minutes for a firmer yolk.

Meanwhile, melt the coconut oil in a skillet over a medium heat and add the cabbage and carrot, sautéing until soft (5-6 minutes).

Add the sesame oil, sautéing for a further 5 minutes and add the green onions at the last minute.

Serve the cabbage in bowls and add the peeled and halved boiled eggs before seasoning with black pepper.

BURRITO BRUNCH

SERVES 2   PREP TIME: 5 MINUTES   COOK TIME: 20 MINUTES

Marvellously Mexican!

- 2 CLOVES GARLIC
- 2 TBSP EXTRA VIRGIN OLIVE OIL
- 1 TBSP CHIPOTLE CHILI POWDER
- 1 TBSP APPLE CIDER VINEGAR
- JUICE OF 1 LIME
- 2 TSP PEPPER
- 1 TSP PAPRIKA
- 1/2 TSP OREGANO
- 2 SKINLESS CHICKEN BREASTS

CILANTRO QUINOA:
- 2 CUPS QUINOA
- JUICE OF 1 LIME
- JUICE OF 1/2 LEMON
- 2 TBSP CHOPPED CILANTRO
- 1/2 ICEBERG OR EQUIVALENT LETTUCE, (SHREDDED FOR SERVING)
- 1 BEEF TOMATO CHOPPED

Take the garlic, chipotle powder, vinegar, lime juice, olive oil, salt, pepper, paprika and the oregano and blend in a blender or pestle and mortar.

Marinate the chicken in this mix for as long as possible.

Heat the broiler to a medium high heat.

Grill the chicken for 10-15 minutes (turning half way through) or until cooked through.

Remove and chop the chicken into cubes.

Meanwhile, boil a pan of water on a medium to high heat and add quinoa before covering and turning down the heat. Allow to simmer for 15-20 minutes with the lid on. Check its fully cooked (it will have soaked up most the water and turned translucent).

Serve quinoa with the oil, lime, lemon juices and chicken and shredded lettuce and tomatoes on top.

Sprinkle with cilantro and enjoy!

PALEO-FRIENDLY ITALIAN OPEN SANDWICH

SERVES 2   PREP TIME: 5 MINUTES   COOK TIME: 30 MINUTES

Choose lean meats for your Italian Panini
and enjoy a taste of the Mediterranean.

---

2 SKINLESS CHICKEN OR TURKEY BREASTS	2 SLICES OF LOW FAT MOZZARELLA (LEAVE IF DAIRY FREE)
2 SLICES OF 100% WHOLEGRAIN BREAD (FRESH NOT PACKAGED)	1/2 TSP BALSAMIC VINEGAR
	1/2 TSP EXTRA VIRGIN OLIVE OIL
1 BEEF TOMATO	1 CUP CHOPPED BASIL
1/2 CUP OF SPINACH	1/2 CUP PINE NUTS
	BLACK PEPPER TO TASTE

Preheat the oven to 375°F/190°C/Gas Mark 5.

Season chicken breasts with a little salt and pepper and wrap in baking/parchment paper.

Bake in the oven for 25-30 minutes or until cooked through.

Meanwhile, prepare the pesto by blending the basil, spinach and pine nuts in a blender or pestle and mortar with the olive oil and balsamic vinegar. Add a little water to loosen the mixture if needed. (Try using walnuts and/or almonds in the pesto if pine nuts are not available).

When chicken ready, toast the wholegrain bread under a broiler for a few minutes until golden.

Layer the bread with sliced tomato, mozzarella and chicken.

Sprinkle with pepper and serve with extra raw spinach leaves and pesto dressing to taste.

LEMON CHICKEN & KOHLRABI SALAD

SERVES 2   PREP TIME: 10 MINUTES   COOK TIME: 10-15 MINUTES

Mouthwatering!

---

2 BONELESS, SKINLESS CHICKEN BREAST HALVES

1 TBSP OF PARSLEY, FRESHLY CHOPPED

2 TBSP. FRESHLY SQUEEZED LEMON JUICE

FOR THE MARINADE:

1 TBSP TURMERIC

1/4 TSP CUMIN

1/2 TSP GINGER, GRATED
SPRINKLE OF GROUND PEPPER

1 TSP EXTRA VIRGIN OLIVE OIL

1/4 CUP WATER

FOR THE SALAD:

1/2 CUCUMBER, DICED

1 CUP WATERCRESS OR RAW SPINACH

1/2 CUP KOHLRABI, THINLY SLICED

Combine the ingredients for the marinade before adding the chicken and covering. If time allows, marinate for one hour up to overnight but don't worry if you need to cook right away!

Preheat broiler to a medium heat and grease a baking tray with olive oil. Shake off the excess marinade from the chicken and then grill for 10 minutes (turning once half way). Check the meat is cooked and piping hot in the middle before removing from broiler and placing to one side.

Carefully slice chicken.

Meanwhile layer the salad onto serving plates and squeeze over the juice of your lemon.

Add finely chopped parsley to serve.

QUINOA WITH CUCUMBER & MINT

SERVES 2 / PREP TIME: 10 MINUTES / COOK TIME: 15 MINUTES

Great for brunch or as a side.

- 1/2 ONION, PEELED AND CHOPPED
- 1 TSP GARLIC, PEELED AND MINCED
- 2 TBSP COCONUT OIL
- 1 TBSP CURRY POWDER
- 1 TSP CUMIN
- 1/2 TSP TURMERIC
- 1 TBSP CILANTRO
- 1 CUP QUINOA
- 1/2 CUCUMBER, DICED
- 1 SPRIG OF FRESH MINT, RIPPED INTO SMALL PIECES WITH YOUR FINGERS
- 1/2 FRESH LEMON

Add the quinoa to a pan of cold water over a high heat.

Allow to boil before covering, lowering the heat and allowing to simmer for 20 minutes or until the water has been soaked up.

Meanwhile, heat the oil in a skillet over a medium-low heat. Sweat the onion and garlic for 3-4 minutes, stirring until softened.

Add the curry powder and cumin to the onions and cook for about 2 minutes, whilst stirring as you smell the beautiful release of flavors!

Add the rest of the cilantro and spices.

For the dressing: Meanwhile prepare the topping by stirring together the cucumber, mint, and juice of ½ lemon.

Mix the dressing through the quinoa and serve.

You can add low fat Greek yogurt to the dressing if your diet allows.

MINTY LAMB STEAK WRAPS

SERVES 2 / PREP TIME: 10 MINUTES / COOK TIME: 25 MINUTES

Juicy and delicious.

- 10 OZ OF LEAN LAMB, CUT INTO STRIPS
- 1 LARGE WHITE ONION, DICED
- 1 CLOVES OF GARLIC, DICED
- 1 TBSP MINT, CHOPPED
- 1 TSP EXTRA VIRGIN OLIVE OIL
- HANDFUL OF PEA SHOOTS OR CRESS
- 4 LARGE ICEBERG, ROMAINE, OR LETTUCE LEAVES FOR THE WRAPS

Heat 1 tsp oil in a pan on a high heat, and then add the lamb and cook for 12-15 minutes or until thoroughly cooked through.

In a separate pan, heat 1 tsp oil and add in the garlic, olive oil and mint to the mix and stir.

Remove from the heat and layer your ingredients inside the lettuce leaf.

Sprinkle over the pea shoots/cress before wrapping the lettuce around the lamb like you would a fajita.

Serve your lettuce wraps warm and enjoy with your hands!

COCONUT SHRIMP

SERVES 2 / PREP TIME: 5 MINUTES / COOK TIME: 20 MINUTES

Fresh and ready in a flash!

- 3 CLOVES OF GARLIC, CRUSHED
- 1 TBSP COCONUT OIL
- 12 JUMBO SHRIMPS
- 1 GREEN ONION, FINELY SLICED
- 1 ZUCCHINI, SPIRALIZED OR CUT INTO THIN STRIPS
- 1 RED BELL PEPPER, SPIRALIZED OR CUT INTO THIN STRIPS

- 1/2 LEMON
- (FOR THE SEASONING)
- DASH OF CHILLI FLAKES
- 1 TBSP COCONUT OIL

Combine the ingredients for the seasoning in a bowl and then add the shrimp and coat.

Heat the coconut oil and garlic in a pan on a medium to high heat, and then add the onion, sautéing for 2 minutes.

Add the dressed shrimp and cook until opaque.

Add the zucchini noodles for 3 minutes and saute.

Add to a sealable glass jar and layer red pepper slices on top with the juice of your lemon.

SOUPS & STEWS

GINGER, CARROT & LIME SOUP

SERVES 2   PREP TIME: 5 MINUTES   COOK TIME: 40 MINS

A real zingy soup – great for winter but can be served cooled in the summer too!

- 2 TBSP OLIVE OIL
- 1 TSP MUSTARD SEEDS, GROUND
- 1 TSP CORIANDER SEEDS, GROUND
- 1 TSP CURRY POWDER
- 1 TBSP GINGER, MINCED
- 4 CUPS CARROTS, THINLY SLICED
- 2 CUPS ONIONS, CHOPPED
- ZEST AND JUICE OF 1 LIME
- 4 CUPS LOW-SALT VEGETABLE BROTH
- BLACK PEPPER FOR TASTE

In a pan on a medium heat, heat the oil, and add the seeds and curry powder for 1 minute.

Add the ginger and then cook for another minute.

Then add in the carrots, onions, and the lime zest, cooking for at least 2 minutes or until the vegetables are soft.

Add the broth and allow to boil before turning heat down slightly and allowing to simmer for 30 minutes.

Allow to cool.

Put the mixture in a food processor and puree until smooth.

Serve with lime juice and black pepper.

ASIAN SQUASH & SHITAKE SOUP

SERVES 2   PREP TIME: 10 MINUTES   COOK TIME: 45 MINS

Chinese mushrooms can be enjoyed endlessly on the anti-inflammatory diet and make a delicious soup.

- 15 DRIED SHIITAKE MUSHROOMS, SOAKED IN WATER
- 6 CUPS LOW SALT VEGETABLE STOCK
- 1/2 BUTTERNUT SQUASH, PEELED AND CUBED
- 1 TBSP SESAME OIL
- 1 ONION, QUARTERED AND SLICED INTO RINGS
- 1 LARGE GARLIC CLOVE, CHOPPED
- 4 STEMS OF PAK CHOY OR EQUIVALENT
- 1 SPRIG OF THYME OR 1 TBSP. DRIED THYME
- 1 TSP TABASCO SAUCE (OPTIONAL)

Heat sesame oil in a large pan on a medium high heat before sweating the onions and garlic.

Add the vegetable stock and bring to a boil over a high heat before adding the squash. Turn down heat and allow to simmer for 25-30 minutes.

Soak the mushrooms in the water if not already done, and then press out the liquid and add to the stock into the pot.

Use the mushroom water in the stock for extra taste.

Add the rest of the ingredients except for the greens and allow to simmer for a further 15 minutes or until the squash is tender.

Add in the chopped greens and let them wilt before serving. Serve with the tabasco sauce if you like it spicy.

SPICED RED PEPPER & TOMATO SOUP

SERVES 2   PREP TIME: 2 MINUTES   COOK TIME: 30 MINS

Hot and Spicy.

---

2 RED BELL PEPPERS

4 BEEF TOMATOES

1 SWEET ONION, CHOPPED

1 GARLIC CLOVE, CHOPPED

3 CUPS HOMEMADE CHICKEN BROTH (SEE RECIPE IN LUNCH SECTION)

2 HABANERO CHILIS WITH THE STEMS REMOVED AND CHOPPED

2 TBSP OF EXTRA VIRGIN OLIVE OIL

Preheat the broiler to a medium high heat and grill the bell peppers, turning half way until the skins are blackened for 10 minutes.

Meanwhile, heat water in a pan on a medium to high heat and cut a small x at the bottom of each tomato using a sharp knife.

Transfer peppers once cooked to a separate dish and cover.

Blanch the tomatoes in simmering water for about 20 seconds.

Remove and plunge into ice cold water.

Peel and chop tomatoes, reserving the juices.

Saute the onion, garlic, chils and 2 tbsp of oil in a saucepan on a medium high heat, stirring until golden for 8-10 minutes.

Add the tomatoes with the juices, the peppers and broth to the onions and cover and simmer for 10-15 minutes or until heated through.

Puree in a blender and serve.

TASTY THAI BROTH

SERVES 2   PREP TIME: 5 MINUTES   COOK TIME: 25 MINUTES

The taste of Thailand can easily be conjured with this fresh and zesty dish.

- 2 TBSP OLIVE OIL
- 1 TBSP SESAME OIL
- 1 TBSP CILANTRO SEEDS
- 1 RED CHILI, FINELY CHOPPED
- A HANDFUL OF FRESH BASIL LEAVES
- 2 SKINLESS COD PIECES
- 2 FRESH LIMES
- 1 GARLIC CLOVE
- 1 THUMB SIZE PIECE OF MINCED GINGER
- 1 WHITE ONION, CHOPPED
- 2 HANDFULS BABY SPINACH LEAVES
- 1 PAC CHOI (LEAVES PULLED OFF SEPARATELY BUT NOT SLICED)
- 1/2 CUP OF HOMEMADE CHICKEN BROTH
- 1/2 CUP OF COCONUT MILK
- 1 RED CHILI, FINELY CHOPPED

Crush the cilantro seeds, chili and basil in a blender or pestle and mortar.

Mix in 1 tbsp of olive oil until a paste is formed.

Heat a large pan/wok with sesame oil on a high heat.

Fry the onions, garlic and ginger for 5-6 minutes until soft but not crispy or browned.

Add the spice paste with the coconut milk into the pan and stir.

Slowly add the stock until a broth is formed.

Now add your fish pieces and allow to simmer in the broth for 10-15 minutes or until cooked through.

Add the pak choi, basil and spinach 2-3 minutes before the end of the cooking time.

Serve with the fresh lime wedges.

MOROCCAN SPICED LENTIL SOUP

SERVES 2   PREP TIME: 5 MINUTES   COOK TIME: 40 MINUTES

Lentils are rich in folic acid and can be enjoyed up to twice a day. They are delicious in this Moroccan inspired soup.

2 TBSP EXTRA VIRGIN OLIVE OIL	2 TBSP LOW FAT GREEK YOGURT
1 YELLOW ONION, DICED	1/2 TSP GROUND TURMERIC
1 CARROTS, DICED	1/2 TSP RED CHILI FLAKES
1 CLOVES OF MINCED GARLIC, DICED	1 CAN CHOPPED TOMATOES
1 TSP GROUND CUMIN	1 CUP DRIED YELLOW LENTILS, SOAKED
1/2 TSP GROUND GINGER	5 CUPS OF LOW SALT VEGETABLE STOCK OR HOMEMADE CHICKEN STOCK
	1 LEMON

In a large pan, heat the oil on a medium high heat.

Sauté the onion and carrot for 5-6 minutes, until softened and starting to brown.

Add the garlic, ginger, chili flakes, cumin and turmeric, cooking for 2 minutes.

Add the tomatoes, scraping any brown bits from the bottom of the pan and cooking until the liquid is reduced (15-20 minutes).

Add the lentils and stock and turn the heat up to reach a boil before lowering heat, covering and then simmering for 10 minutes.

Serve with a wedge of lemon on the side and a dollop of Greek yogurt.

FLAVERSOME VEGETARIAN TAGINE

SERVES 2   PREP TIME: 10 MINUTES   COOK TIME: 35 MINUTES

A vegetarian take on this Moroccan classic.

- 2 TBSP COCONUT OIL
- 1 ONION, DICED
- 1 PARSNIP, PEELED AND DICED
- 2 CLOVES OF GARLIC
- 1 TSP GROUND CUMIN
- 1/2 TSP GROUND GINGER
- 1/2 TSP GROUND CINNAMON
- 1/4 TSP CAYENNE PEPPER
- 3 TBSP TOMATO PASTE
- 1 SWEET POTATO, PEELED & DICED
- 1 PURPLE POTATO, PEELED & DICED
- 4 BABY CARROTS, PEELED & DICED
- 4 CUPS LOW-SALT VEGETABLE STOCK
- 2 CUPS KALE LEAVES
- 2 TBSP LEMON JUICE
- 1/4 CUP CILANTRO, ROUGHLY CHOPPED
- HANDFUL OF TOASTED ALMONDS

In a large pot, heat the oil on a medium high heat before sautéing the onion until soft.

Add the parsnip for 10 minutes or until golden brown.

Add the garlic, cumin, ginger, cinnamon, tomato paste, and cayenne.

Cook for about 2 minutes until the lovely scents reach your nose.

Fold in the sweet potatoes, carrots, and the purple potatoes and stock and then bring to a boil.

Turn heat down and simmer for 20 minutes.

Add in the kale and lemon juice, simmering for a further 2 minutes or until the leaves are slightly wilted.

Garnish with the cilantro and the nuts to serve.

WINTER WARMING CHUNKY CHICKEN SOUP

SERVES 4   PREP TIME: 7 MINUTES   COOK TIME: 40 MINS

Nostalgic and homemade – beats inflammation and warms the soul!

---

1 WHOLE FREE RANGE CHICKEN (NO GIBLETS), COOKED

1 BAY LEAF

5 CUPS OF HOMEMADE CHICKEN BROTH/WATER

1 ONION, CHOPPED

2 STALKS OF CELERY, SLICED

3 CARROTS, CHOPPED AND PEELED

2 PARSNIPS, CHOPPED AND PEELED

SPRINKLE OF PEPPER TO SEASON

Add all of the ingredients minus the pepper into a large pot and boil on a high heat.

Once boiling, lower the heat and allow to simmer for 30 minutes, or until the chicken is piping hot throughout.

Remove the chicken and place on a chopping board.

Slice as much meat as you can from the chicken and remove the skin and bones.

Add it back into the pot and either serve right away as a chunky soup or allow to cool and whizz through the blender to serve.

Add black pepper to season and serve alone or with your choice of wholegrain bread – quinoa tastes delicious with this too – just pop it into the soup 20 minutes before the end and it will soak up all the delicious flavors.

Top tip: If you have leftovers, strain and keep in a sealed container as chicken broth. You can keep this for 2-3 days in the fridge or 3-4 weeks in the freezer.

CURRIED LENTIL & SPINACH STEW

SERVES 2   PREP TIME: 5 MINUTES   COOK TIME: 30 MINUTES

A hearty and wholesome stew with the flavors of India.

- 1 TBSP EXTRA-VIRGIN OLIVE OIL
- 1 TBSP CURRY POWDER
- 1 CUP HOMEMADE CHICKEN OR VEGETABLE STOCK
- 1 CUP RED LENTILS, SOAKED
- 1 ONION, CHOPPED
- 2 CUPS BUTTERNUT SQUASH, COOKED PEELED AND CHOPPED
- 1 CUP SPINACH
- 2 GARLIC CLOVES, MINCED
- 1 TBSP CILANTRO, FINELY CHOPPED

In a large pot, add the oil, chopped onion and minced garlic, sautéing for 5 minutes on low heat.

Add the curry powder and ginger to the onions and cook for 5 minutes.

Add the broth and bring to a boil on a high heat.

Stir in the lentils, squash and spinach, reduce heat and simmer for a further 20 minutes.

Season with pepper to taste and serve with fresh cilantro.

CILANTRO & CARROT SOUP

SERVES 2   PREP TIME: 5 MINUTES   COOK TIME: 40 MINS

Serve hot or cold!

- 2 TBSP OLIVE OIL
- 1 TSP CILANTRO SEEDS, GROUND
- 1 TSP CURRY POWDER
- 1 TBSP GINGER, MINCED
- 4 CUPS CARROTS, THINLY SLICED
- 2 CUPS ONIONS, CHOPPED
- ZEST AND JUICE OF 1 LIME
- 2 TBSP FRESH CILANTRO TO SERVE
- 4 CUPS LOW-SALT/HOMEMADE VEGETABLE BROTH
- BLACK PEPPER FOR TASTE

In a pan on a medium heat, heat the oil, and add the seeds and curry powder for 1 minute.

Add the ginger and then cook for another minute.

Then add in the carrots, onions, and the lime zest, cooking for at least 2 minutes or until the vegetables are soft.

Add the broth and allow to boil before turning heat down slightly and allowing to simmer for 30 minutes. Allow to cool.

Put the mixture in a food processor and puree until smooth.
Serve with lime juice, fresh cilantro and black pepper.

PUMPKIN & PARSLEY SOUP

SERVES 2   PREP TIME: 10 MINUTES   COOK TIME: 45 MINS

Winter warmer!

1/2 PUMPKIN

3 CUPS LOW SALT/HOMEMADE VEGETABLE STOCK

1 TBSP SESAME OIL

1 ONION, QUARTERED AND SLICED INTO RINGS

1 LARGE GARLIC CLOVE, CHOPPED

1/2 CUP FRESH PARSLEY

1 THUMB SIZED PIECE OF GINGER, GRATED

Prepare the pumpkin by removing the top with a sharp knife and scooping out the flesh from the inside.

Remove the seeds, wash and place to one side.

Heat sesame oil in a large pan on a medium high heat before sweating the onions and garlic.

Add the vegetable stock and bring to a boil over a high heat before adding the pumpkin flesh.

Add the parsley and ginger and stir.

Turn down heat and allow to simmer for 40-45 minutes.

Whizz up in a blender and serve hot with the pumpkin seeds scattered over the top to serve.

HOMEMADE VEGETABLE STOCK

SERVES 2   PREP TIME: 10 MINUTES   COOK TIME: 35 MINUTES

A simple stock recipe for use in many of the recipes in this cookbook.

2 ONIONS	1 TBSP EXTRA VIRGIN OLIVE OIL
3 CARROTS	1 BAY LEAF
3 CELERY STALKS	1 TBSP THYME
1 GARLIC CLOVE	1 TBSP PARSLEY
	1 TSP BLACK PEPPERCORNS

Peel and chop vegetables and soak in warm water.

Heat the oil in a large pot over a medium heat and add the vegetables, garlic, herbs and peppercorns, cooking for 5 minutes.

Fill up the pot with boiling water.

Turn up the heat and bring to the boil - allow to simmer for 25 minutes.

Strain stock and use immediately or allow to cool and refrigerate for 2-3 days or freeze for 3-4 weeks in a sealed container.

HOMEMADE HEALTHY CHICKEN STOCK

SERVES 2   PREP TIME: 10 MINUTES   COOK TIME: 4 HOURS

This homemade chicken stock is far healthier than shop bought and can be used in some of the recipes featured in this cookbook. It's delicious too.

- 1 WHOLE ROASTING CHICKEN {AROUND 4-5LBS}
- 3 CARROTS, SOAKED IN WARM WATER
- 2 MEDIUM ONIONS
- 4 GARLIC CLOVES, CRUSHED
- 2 BAY LEAVES
- 3 STALKS OF CELERY, SOAKED IN WARM WATER
- 1 TBSP EACH DRIED ROSEMARY, THYME, PEPPER, TURMERIC
- 1 TBSP WHITE WINE VINEGAR
- 11-12 CUPS WATER

Rinse off your chicken and place in a large saucepan or soup pan (remove giblets but don't waste them; add them in to your stock bowl!)

Chop your vegetables into large chunks (quarters at the smallest). Leave the skins on as they add to the taste and the nutrients - add to the pan.

Add the herbs, spices and pepper to the pan.

Fill your pan with water so that the chicken and vegetables are completely covered.

Turn stove on high and bring to boiling point before reducing the heat and allowing the stock to simmer for 3-4 hours.

Check at intervals and top up with water if the ingredients become uncovered. Take off the heat and carefully remove the chicken, placing to one side.

You now need to strain the liquid from the stockpot into another bowl using a sieve to get rid of all the lumpy bits.

Leave the stock and chicken to cool.

Once cool, tear or cut the meat from the bones.

Once the stock has cooled to room temperature, add to a sealed container and keep in the fridge.

MIXED BEAN SPICY SOUP

SERVES 2   PREP TIME: 5 MINUTES   COOK TIME: 40 MINUTES

A little kick to a nutritious soup.

- 2 TBSP EXTRA VIRGIN OLIVE OIL
- 1 ONION, DICED
- 1 CLOVE OF MINCED GARLIC, DICED
- 1 TSP GROUND CUMIN
- 1/2 TSP GROUND GINGER
- 1/2 TSP GROUND TURMERIC
- 1/2 TSP RED CHILI FLAKES
- 1/4 CUP DRIED KIDNEY LENTILS, SOAKED
- 1/4 CUP LIMA BEANS
- 5 CUPS OF HOMEMADE VEGETABLE STOCK OR HOMEMADE CHICKEN STOCK
- 1 LEMON

In a large pan, heat the oil on a medium to high heat.

Sauté the onion for 5-6 minutes, until softened and starting to brown.

Add the garlic, ginger, chili flakes, cumin and turmeric, cooking for 2 minutes.

Add the stock, lentils and beans and turn the heat up to reach boiling point before lowering heat, covering and simmering for 30 minutes.

Serve with a wedge of lemon on the side.

CHICKEN & LENTIL SOUP

SERVES 2   PREP TIME: 7 MINUTES   COOK TIME: 50 MINS

A delicious cold-busting chicken soup.

---

1 WHOLE FREE RANGE CHICKEN (NO GIBLETS), COOKED

1 BAY LEAF

5 CUPS OF HOMEMADE CHICKEN BROTH/WATER

1 ONION, CHOPPED

2 STALKS OF CELERY, SLICED

3 CARROTS, CHOPPED AND PEELED

2 TURNIPS, CHOPPED AND PEELED

SPRINKLE OF PEPPER TO SEASON

1/2 CUP KIDNEY LENTILS, SOAKED

Add all of the ingredients minus the pepper into a large pot and boil on a high heat.

Once boiling, lower the heat and allow to simmer for 30 minutes, or until the chicken is piping hot throughout.

Remove the chicken and place on a chopping board.

Slice as much meat as you can from the chicken and remove the skin and bones.

Add it back into the pot with the quinoa and allow to cook for a further 20 minutes.

Serve right away as a chunky soup.

Add black pepper to season and serve.

Top tip: If you have leftovers, strain and keep in a sealed container as chicken broth. You can keep this for 2-3 days in the fridge or 3-4 weeks in the freezer.

KALE & SWEET POTATO SOUP

SERVES 2   PREP TIME: 5 MINUTES   COOK TIME: 30 MINUTES

Packed full of flavor!

---

1 TBSP EXTRA-VIRGIN OLIVE OIL	1 ONION, CHOPPED
1 TSP TURMERIC	4 CUPS SPINACH
1 TSP CUMIN	2 GARLIC CLOVES, MINCED
1 CUP HOMEMADE CHICKEN OR VEGETABLE STOCK	
2 SWEET POTATOES, PEELED & CHOPPED	

In a large pot, add the oil, chopped onion and minced garlic, sautéing for 5 minutes on low heat.

Add the spices to the onions and cook for 5 minutes.

Add the broth and bring to a boil on a high heat.

Stir in the sweet potatoes, reduce heat and simmer for a further 20 minutes.

Add the spinach in the last 5 minutes to wilt.

Season with pepper and serve as a chunky soup or whizz up in a blender for a smooth soup.

SMOOTHIES AND DRINKS

GINGERY GREEN ICED-TEA

SERVES 1   PREP TIME: 5 MINUTES   COOK TIME: NA

A refreshing iced-tea with anti-inflammatory properties.

---

2 CUPS CONCENTRATED GREEN OR MACHA TEA, SERVED HOT

1/4 CUP CRYSTALIZED GINGER, CHOPPED INTO FINE PIECES

1 SPRIG OF FRESH MINT

Get a glass container and mix the tea with the ginger and then cover and chill for as long as time permits.

Strain and pour into serving glasses over ice if you wish.

Garnish with a wedge of lemon and a sprig of fresh mint to serve.

MULTI-VITAMIN SMOOTHIE

SERVES 1   PREP TIME: 5 MINUTES   COOK TIME: NA

This delectable smoothie is full of powerful antioxidants.

---

1 CUP RED OR WHITE GRAPES	1/2 CUP ICE CUBES
1 CUP SLICED FROZEN OR FRESH PEACHES	1/2 CUP WATER
1 CUP CHOPPED CABBAGE	1 SPRIG OF FRESH MINT
1 CARROT, PEELED AND SLICED	

Toss all of the ingredients in a blender or juicer until smooth.

Serve immediately in a tall glass with fresh mint to garnish.

BANANA & APPLE BLEND

SERVES 1   PREP TIME: 5 MINUTES   COOK TIME: NA

A breakfast or snack– this tastes excellent and keeps you going until your next meal.

1 BANANA	2 CUPS FILTERED WATER
1 APPLE, CORED AND PEELED	1 TBSP STEVIA
2 TBSP FLAXSEED OIL	1 CUP LOW FAT COCONUT MILK
2 TBSP WHOLE OAT BRAN	1 CUP OF SPINACH OR EQUIVALENT GREEN OF YOUR CHOICE

In a food processor, add all of the ingredients except for the greens, processing until smooth.

Mix in the greens and then blend until smooth.

Serve over ice.

BLUEBERRY AND SPINACH SHAKE

SERVES 1   PREP TIME: 2 MINUTES   COOK TIME: NA

We eat with our eyes and this shake looks deliciously purple when first prepared. It's packed with antioxidants and iron.

- 1 CUP OF LOW FAT GREEK YOGURT (OPTIONAL)
- 1 CUP ORGANIC BLUEBERRIES (OR WASHED IF NON-ORGANIC)
- 1/2 CUP SPINACH
- ICE CUBES TO DESIRED CONCENTRATION

Add ingredients together in a blender until smooth and then serve in a tall glass.

Sprinkle a few fresh berries on top if you wish!

ANTIOXIDANT SMOOTHIE

SERVES 1   PREP TIME: 2 MINUTES   COOK TIME: NA

Great for boosting brain power and reducing inflammation at the same time.

- 1 CUP FROZEN BLUEBERRIES
- 1/2 BANANA
- 1/2 CUP CUCUMBER, CHOPPED
- 1 TBSP FLAXSEEDS
- 1 CUP COCONUT WATER

Take all of the ingredients and blend until smooth.

You can add ice cubes at this point if you want it chilled.

Serve.

SYMPTOM SOOTHING SMOOTHIE

SERVES 1   PREP TIME: 2 MINUTES   COOK TIME: NA

An immediate pain relief for when your symptoms flare up.

---

1 STALK CELERY, CHOPPED	1/2 LEMON, ZEST JUICE
1 CUP CUCUMBER, CHOPPED	1 CUP COCONUT WATER
1/2 CUP PINEAPPLE, CHOPPED	1 APPLE, CHOPPED

Take all of the ingredients (minus the lemon zest) and blend until smooth.

You can add ice cubes at this point if you want it chilled.

Serve with a sprinkling of lemon zest.

WONDERFUL WATERMELON DRINK

SERVES 1   PREP TIME: 2 MINUTES   COOK TIME: NA

This is a great fruit juice packed with an array of vitamins.

- 1 CUP WATERMELON CHUNKS
- 2 CUPS FROZEN MIXED BERRIES
- 1 CUP COCONUT WATER
- 2 TBSP CHIA SEEDS
- 1/2 CUP OF TART CHERRIES

Blend ingredients in a blender or juicer until pureed.

Serve immediately and enjoy!

SWEET & SAVOURY SMOOTHIE

SERVES 1   PREP TIME: 10 MINUTES   COOK TIME: NA

The spices used in this smoothie make it fantastic for anti-inflammatory purposes but also a more savory drink between meals.

- 2 CUPS CARROTS, PEELED AND SLICED
- 2 CUPS FILTERED WATER.
- 1 APPLE, PEELED AND SLICED
- 1 BANANA, PEELED AND SLICED
- 1 CUP FRESH PINEAPPLE, PEELED AND SLICED
- 1/2 TBSP GINGER, GRATED
- 1/4 TSP GROUND TURMERIC
- 1 TBSP LEMON JUICE
- 1 CUP ALMOND OR SOY MILK

Blend carrots and water to make a pureed carrot juice.

Pour into a Mason jar or sealable container, cover and place in fridge.

Once done, add the rest of the smoothie ingredients to a blender or juicer until smooth.

Add the carrot juice in at the end, blending thoroughly until smooth.

Serve with or without ice.

BLACKBERRY & GINGER MILKSHAKE

SERVES 1   PREP TIME: 2 MINUTES   COOK TIME: NA

Inflammation combating and delightful.

- 1 THUMB SIZED PIECE OF GINGER, GRATED
- 2 CUPS BLACKBERRIES, WASHED
- 2 CUPS CHOPPED PEACHES
- 2 CUPS ALMOND MILK

Add all the ingredients to a blender or juicer and blend together until smooth.

Serve with a scattering of fresh blackberries and enjoy!

ALMOND & TURMERIC CHAI TEA

SERVES 4   PREP TIME: 2 MINUTES   COOK TIME: 2 MINUTES

A timeless healer, turmeric is used for its anti-inflammatory properties and makes a delicious chai!

- 3 TBSP TURMERIC
- 4 TSP CINNAMON
- 1/8 TSP GROUND CLOVES
- 1 TSP GROUND CARDAMOM
- 1 TSP GROUND GINGER
- 1 TSP CAYENNE PEPPER
- 4 TSP CHAI TEA POWDER
- 4 CUPS BOILING WATER
- HONEY TO TASTE
- 1 CUP ALMOND MILK

Combine all of the ingredients excluding the milk and honey in a glass container, mix well and then seal.

Pour boiling water into 2 tbsp of the tea mix (use a tea strainer to serve).

You can then add almond milk and honey to taste.

Save the tea mix in a sealed container, storing in a dry place for future chais!

HOMEMADE APPLE TEA

SERVES 4   PREP TIME: OVERNIGHT   COOK TIME: 0 MINUTES

If you like something a little more sweet, this apple-infusion is perfect for you.

- 4 CUPS BOILING WATER
- 4 TBSP FRESH GREEN TEA LEAVES
- 5 APPLES, PEELED AND SLICED.
- 1 TSP CINNAMON

Pour boiling water over tea leaves through a tea strainer, allowing to steep for 5 minutes.

Add the apple slices and cinnamon to the boiling water and transfer into a sealable container.

Chill overnight to allow apple to infuse before serving.

Garnish with fresh apple slices and mint to serve over ice.

FRESH CRANBERRY AND LIME JUICE

SERVES 4   PREP TIME: 5 MINUTES   COOK TIME: 0 MINUTES

An anti-inflammatory blend for your juicer.

---

4 CUPS CRANBERRIES

2 LIMES, JUICED

1/2 CUP SPINACH

1/2 CUP OF MIXED BERRIES (FROZEN ARE FINE)

Mix all the ingredients with water in a juicer until pureed and served immediately over ice.

FRESH TROPICAL JUICE

SERVES 4   PREP TIME: 5 MINUTES   COOK TIME: 30 MINUTES

A Caribbean treat, helping you fight symptoms and continue enjoying sweet drinks.

---

1 WHOLE FRESH PINEAPPLE, PEELED AND CUT INTO CHUNKS.

1/2 CAN LOW FAT COCONUT MILK

1 CUP WATER

Add all ingredients to a juicer and blend until smooth.

Serve over ice.

MIXED FRUIT & NUT MILKSHAKE

SERVES 2   PREP TIME: 5 MINUTES   COOK TIME: 30 MINUTES

This smoothie not only contains the antioxidants found in fruit, but has protein from the nuts too.

1/2 GRAPEFRUIT, PEELED AND CHOPPED	JUICE OF 1 ORANGE
2 TBSP CHOPPED ALMONDS	1 TBSP HONEY
1/2 INCH PIECE OF GINGER, MINCED	1/2 CUP ALMOND MILK
	12 STRAWBERRIES

Put everything but the strawberries in a blender until smooth.

Add in the strawberries and blend until pureed, serving in a tall glass.

SUPER STRAWBERRY SMOOTHIE

SERVES 2   PREP TIME: 5 MINUTES   COOK TIME: 30 MINUTES

A sweet treat to be enjoyed without any guilt!

1 STALK OF CELERY, CHOPPED	1 CUP STRAWBERRIES
1/2 CUP OF KALE	1 LIME WEDGE
1/2 CUP OF SPINACH	1 CUP COCONUT WATER

Take all of the ingredients and blend until smooth.

Serve over ice.

PEACH ICED TEA

SERVES 2   PREP TIME: 5 MINUTES   COOK TIME: NA

A perfect thirst-quencher for you both.

---

2 CUPS CONCENTRATED GREEN OR MACHA TEA, SERVED HOT

1 PEACH, PEELED AND SLICED

2 WEDGES OF LEMON

Get a glass container and mix the tea with the peach slices and then cover and chill for as long as time permits.

Strain and pour into serving glasses over ice if you wish.

Garnish with a wedge of lemon to serve.

STRAWBERRY & MINT SMOOTHIE

SERVES 2   PREP TIME: 5 MINUTES   COOK TIME: NA

This delectable smoothie is full of powerful antioxidants.

- 1 CUP STAWBERRIES
- 1 CUP SLICED FROZEN OR FRESH PEACHES
- 1/2 CUP ICE CUBES
- 1/2 CUP WATER
- 2 TBSP MINT, FINELY CHOPPED
- 1 LIME, JUICED

Toss all of the ingredients in a blender or juicer until smooth.

Serve immediately in a tall glass.

PRETTY PURPLE PUNCH

SERVES 2   PREP TIME: 2 MINUTES   COOK TIME: NA

The blueberries and raspberries turn a delicious purple flavor and are packed with anti inflammatory properties.

- 1 CUP OF LOW FAT GREEK YOGURT/ALMOND MILK
- 1 CUP ORGANIC BLUEBERRIES (OR WASHED IF NON-ORGANIC)
- 1 CUP RASPBERRIES
- ICE CUBES TO DESIRED CONCENTRATION

Add ingredients together in a blender until smooth and then serve in a tall glass.

Sprinkle a few fresh berries on top if you wish!

ALMOND & CRANBERRY SHAKE

SERVES 2   PREP TIME: 5 MINUTES   COOK TIME: 30 MINUTES

A healthy milkshake!

- 4 TBSP CHOPPED ALMONDS
- 1/2 CUP CRANBERRIES
- 1 TBSP RAW HONEY
- 1 CUP ALMOND MILK

Blend and serve over ice!

BEEF AND PORK MAIN DISHES

HERBY CHUCK ROAST & SCRUMMY VEG

SERVES 4   PREP TIME: 10 MINUTES   COOK TIME: 7 HOURS IN CROCK POT

This is an awesome meal to be shared with the family!

- 16 OZ OF LEAN CHUCK ROAST
- 1 TSP PEPPER
- 2 ONIONS CUT, PEELED AND QUARTERED
- 8 BABY CARROTS, PEELED AND QUARTED
- 1 STALK OF CELERY, SLICED
- 1 BAY LEAF
- 10 CUPS WATER
- 1 CAULIFLOWER, CUT INTO FLORETS
- 5 CHERRY TOMATOES

SEASONING:
- 1 TBSP CAYENNE PEPPER
- 2 TBSP DRIED/FRESH ROSEMARY

Use a sharp knife to trim any fat from the chuck roast.

Season the meat with the herbs and spices.

Put the onions, carrots, and celery into the crock pot/slow cooker, then the meat, and finally add the bay leaf and water.

Cook on low for about 5-7 hours or until the meat is tender.

You can then add the cauliflower and cherry tomatoes for the last 15 minutes or until cooked through.

Serve hot.

FAST AND FRESH LEAN BEEF BURGERS

SERVES 2   PREP TIME: 5 MINUTES   COOK TIME: 25 MINUTES

Yes you can still enjoy a burger from time to time!

- 8 OZ OF LEAN 100% GRASS-FED GROUND BEEF
- 1 TSP BLACK PEPPER
- 1 TSP GARLIC POWDER
- 1 TSP COCONUT OIL
- 1 ONION, SLICED
- 1 AVOCADO, SLICED
- 2 TBSP BALSAMIC VINEGAR
- 1 LARGE TOMATO CUT INTO 6 SLICES

Mix the ground beef with the pepper and garlic powder.

Heat a skillet on a medium to high heat, and then add the coconut oil.

Sauté the onions for 5-10 minutes until browned.

Then add in the balsamic vinegar and sauté for another 5 minutes.

Form burger shapes with the ground beef using the palms of your hands, add to the skillet and sauté on each side for about 5-6 minutes. Remove.

Let them sit on a tray to cool slightly and then assemble your burger on your serving plate by adding your sliced tomato, avocado and onions on the top.

You can serve as a bunless burger with salad or with a 100% wholegrain burger bun as you choose.

MAKE YOUR OWN PIZZA

SERVES 4   PREP TIME: 10 MINUTES   COOK TIME: 40 MINUTES

If you thought you had to give up pizza then you can think again!

FOR THE BASE:

1 CUP TAPIOCA STARCH

1/2 CUP COCONUT FLOUR

2 FREE RANGE EGGS

1 CUP WATER

FOR THE TOPPING:

1/2 CAN CHOPPED TOMATOES

1 CLOVE GARLIC, MINCED

1 SPRIG ROSEMARY

1 SPRIG BASIL

2 BEEF TOMATOES, SLICED

1 JALAPENO, SLICED

1/2 CUP WATERCRESS OR SPINACH

1 ONION, CHOPPED

1/2 CUP LEAN MEAT OF YOUR CHOICE, COOKED AND SLICED

Heat oven to 375°f/190°c/Gas Mark 5.

Get a bowl and mix together all of the ingredients for the base until a smooth dough is formed, adding a little more water if necessary.

Roll the dough into a pizza base (don't worry if it's not perfect!)

Sauté onions and garlic over a medium heat and add chopped tomatoes and herbs, cooking for 5-10 minutes.

Layer the base with the tomato sauce, jalapeno, herbs, tomato slices and meat pieces and then bake in the oven for 30 minutes on a slatted rack.

Ensure the base is cooked through and not soggy.

Cut into eights, and then serve immediately with the watercress or spinach scattered on top.

LOVELY LAMB BURGERS & MINTY YOGURT

SERVES 2   PREP TIME: 5 MINUTES   COOK TIME: 20 MINUTES

A lighter alternative to a classic beef burger which tastes delicious with this minty-yogurt dip.

- 8 OZ LEAN GROUND LAMB
- 1 TBSP FRESH ROSEMARY, FINELY CHOPPED
- 1/2 CUP EXTRA VIRGIN OLIVE OIL
- 1 LEMON, JUICED
- 1 CLOVE OF GARLIC, MINCED
- 1/2 CUP OF LOW FAT GREEK YOGURT
- 1/4 CUCUMBER, CHOPPED
- 1/2 BUNCH FRESH MINT
- 1/2 CUP ARUGULA

Mix together the ground lamb, garlic and rosemary and a drizzle of the olive oil until combined, and then shape 1 inch thick patties with your hands.

Heat the rest of the oil in a skillet over a medium-high heat, and then cook the patties for 16 minues, flipping once halfway through and ensuring they are cooked throughout.

Mix the yogurt, lemon juice, mint and cucumber and serve on top of the lamb burger with a side salad of arugula.

Serve warm.

SLOW COOKED BEEF BRISKET

SERVES 4   PREP TIME: 10 MINUTES   COOK TIME: 4 HOURS

Tempting and tender, this is a real treat!

- 16 OZ OF 100 GRASS FED BEEF BRISKET WITH THE FAT TRIMMED
- 2 CLOVES GARLIC, MINCED
- 1 SPRIG OF THYME
- 1 SPRIG OF ROSEMARY
- 1 TBSP MUSTARD
- 1/4 CUP EXTRA VIRGIN OLIVE OIL
- 1/4 TSP GROUND PEPPER
- 1 ONION, SLICED
- 1 CUP CARROTS, SLICED
- 2 CUPS CHOPPED TOMATOES

Heat oven to 300°F/150°C/Gas Mark 2.

Use a fork to make a paste by mashing the mustard, thyme and rosemary with the garlic before mixing in the oil and pepper.

Pour the mixture over the brisket.

Place half of the veggies onto the bottom of a baking dish.

Place the beef on top of the vegetables and cover with the rest of the vegetables and chopped tomatoes.

Bake in the oven or slow cooker for about 3-4 hours, or until tender and serve with your favorite side.

SUPER LAMB SHOULDER WITH APRICOT & ZUCCHINI MASH

SERVES 4   PREP TIME: 5 MINUTES   COOK TIME: 4-5 HOURS

A very quick and easy, healthy lamb recipe to liven up your day!

- 1 LEAN LAMB SHOULDERS
- 2 ZUCCHINIS, CHOPPED
- 4 TBSP. EXTRA VIRGIN OLIVE OIL
- 5 SPRIGS ROSEMARY
- 3 SPRIGS THYME
- 1 TSP BLACK PEPPER
- 1/2 CUP APRICOTS
- HANDFUL OF ARUGULA
- 2 GARLIC CLOVES, CHOPPED
- 8 BABY CHERRY TOMATOES, HALVED
- HANDFUL OF CHOPPED CILANTRO

Preheat oven to its highest setting.

Prepare the meat by trimming the fat layer off.

Rub the lamb with 3 tbsp olive oil, rosemary and thyme as well as a little black pepper.

Line a baking tray with the apricots.

Cover the dish with aluminum foil or a baking lid.

Turn the oven down to 325°f/170°c/Gas Mark 3 and add the lamb.

Cook for 4-5 hours and remove and rest.

Now, add 1 tbsp oil to a pan and heat on a medium heat.

Throw in the zucchinis, tomatoes and garlic and sauté for 5-6 minutes until soft. Add the arugula and cilantro and stir in.

Serve the lamb on a bed of the veg, drizzling over the juices from the bottom of the pan for extra-deliciousness!

CHILI BEEF & BROCCOLI CURRY

SERVES 4   PREP TIME: 2 MINUTES   COOK TIME: 50 MINUTES

Scrumptious curry, so simple to make!

- 16 OZ OF 100% GRASS-FED SIRLOIN OR FILLET STEAK
- 2 TBSP OF COCONUT OIL
- 2 GARLIC CLOVES, MINCED
- 1 TBSP OF LEMON JUICE
- 1 CUP OF HOMEMADE CHICKEN BROTH
- 1 CUP CARROTS, CHOPPED
- 1 ONION, CHOPPED
- 1 RED CHILI, FINELY CHOPPED
- 2 TBSP OF GINGER, GRATED
- 1 TBSP OF BLACK PEPPER
- 1 CUP OF BROCCOLI

Pre-heat the coconut oil and garlic in a large pan over a high heat.

Add the diced steak to the pan and brown both sides for around 5-6 minutes.

Once brown, take the beef out and leave to one side.

Get a bowl and mix the pepper, ginger, lemon juice and ¼ of the homemade chicken broth.

Add the broth mix and the beef back into the pan as well as the chopped onions and chili.

Add the last of the stock over the beef and turn down to a simmer for 40 minutes or until piping hot and beef is cooked through.

When there are only 15-20 minutes left of the cooking time, add the broccoli and chopped carrots into the pan.

Serve right away.

MIGHTY HERB PORK MEATBALLS

SERVES 2   PREP TIME: 5 MINUTES   COOK TIME: 20 MINUTES

These meatballs are made with lean pork so are less inflammatory than beef. They also taste magnificent!

8 OZ LEAN PORK MINCE	FOR THE SAUCE:
1 GARLIC CLOVE, CRUSHED	1 TBSP EXTRA VIRGIN OLIVE OIL
1/4 CUP 100% WHOLEGRAIN BREAD CRUMBS	1 RED ONION, FINELY CHOPPED
1 TSP DRIED THYME	1 CAN CHOPPED TOMATOES
1 TSP DRIED BASIL	1 RED PEPPER (OPTIONAL), FINELY CHOPPED
2 TBSP EXTRA VIRGIN OLIVE OIL	1/2 CUP WATER
1 CUP 100% WHOLEGRAIN OR GLUTEN FREE SPAGHETTI TO SERVE	1 TBSP FRESH BASIL

Mix the pork mince, 1 tbsp oil, garlic, breadcrumbs and herbs in a bowl. Season with a little black pepper and separate into 8 balls, rolling with the palms of your hands.

Heat 1 tbsp oil in a pan over a medium heat and add onions and peppers, sautéing for a few minutes until softened.

Add the tomatoes and ½ cup water.

Cover and lower heat to simmer for 15 minutes.

Meanwhile, boil your water and cook spaghetti to recommended guidelines.

In a separate pan, heat 1 tbsp oil and add the meatballs, turning carefully to brown the surface of each. Continue this for 5-7 minutes before adding to the sauce and simmering for a further 5 minutes.

Drain spaghetti, portion up and pour a generous portion of meatballs and sauce over the top to serve.

Sprinkle with a little freshly torn basil!

THAI BEEF WITH COCONUT MILK

SERVES 2 PREP TIME: 5 MINUTES COOK TIME: 35 MINUTES

Fast and fresh!

- 2 TBSP COCONUT OIL
- 1 TSP CRUSHED GARLIC
- 1 ONION CUT INTO WEDGES
- 8 OZ ROUND STEAK, CUT INTO STRIPS
- 2 SLICED CELERY STALKS
- 1 LIME
- 1 RED CAPSICUM, CUT INTO PIECES
- 1 TBSP RED CHILI FLAKES
- 2 CUPS BROCCOLI FLORETS
- 1 CUP COCONUT MILK
- 1/2 CUP BEEF STOCK
- BLACK PEPPER TO TASTE

Heat the wok over a medium heat, and then add in the oil, garlic, and the onion, cooking for 1 minute.

Put the beef into the wok and cook for 3 minutes.

Add in the celery, broccoli, and capsicum into the wok and stir-fry for 4 minutes.

Add the coconut milk, beef stock, chili flakes and black pepper and allow to simmer for 20-25 minutes or until beef is cooked through.

Serve hot with your choice of greens and a wedge of lime to squeeze!

LUSH LAMB & ROSEMARY CASSEROLE

SERVES 2   PREP TIME: 5 MINUTES   COOK TIME: 1 HOUR 15 MINUTES

Hearty, wholesome and super easy to make!

- 1 TBSP OF OLIVE OIL
- 2 LEAN LAMB FILLETS, CUBED
- 1 ONION, CHOPPED
- 2 CARROTS, CUBED
- 1/2 CUP KALE
- 4 CUPS OF HOMEMADE CHICKEN STOCK
- 1 TSP DRIED ROSEMARY
- 1 TSP OF CHOPPED PARSLEY
- 2 CANS RINSED AND DRAINED CANNELLINI BEANS

In a large casserole dish, heat the olive oil on a medium high heat.

Add the lamb and cook for 5 minutes until browned.

Add the chopped onion and carrots. Leave to cook for another 5 minutes until the vegetables begin to soften.

Add the chicken stock, kale and rosemary.

Then cover the casserole and leave to simmer on a low heat for 1-1.5 hours until the lamb is tender and fully cooked through.

Add the cannellini beans 15 minutes before the end of the cooking time.

Plate up and serve with the chopped parsley to garnish.

BEEF CHILI & QUINOA

SERVES 2   PREP TIME: 10 MINUTES   COOK TIME: 30 MINUTES

A delicious anti inflammatory dish.

---

1 RED ONION, DICED

2 GARLIC CLOVES, MINCED

8 OZ LEAN GROUND BEEF

1 TSP CHILI FLAKES

1 TSP OREGANO

Bring a pan of water to the boil and add quinoa for 20 minutes.

Meanwhile, add the oil to a pan and heat on a medium to high heat.

Add the onions and garlic and sauté for 5 minutes until soft.

Remove and set aside.

Add the beef to the pan and stir until browned.

Add the vegetables back into the pan and stir.

Now add the chili flakes, herbs and tomatoes; cover and turn the heat down a little to simmer for 15 minutes.

Meanwhile, drain the water from the quinoa. Replace the lid and steam while the chili is cooking.

Serve hot with the fresh cilantro sprinkled over the top.

CHINESE STYLE BEEF WRAPS

SERVES 2   PREP TIME: 10 MINUTES   COOK TIME: 30 MINUTES

Fast and fresh!

1 GARLIC CLOVE, MINCED	1 TBSP APPLE CIDER VINEGAR
1/2 CUCUMBER, DICED	1 TSP GROUND GINGER
5 OZ LEAN GROUND BEEF	2 ICEBERG LETTUCE LEAVES
1 TBSP CHILI FLAKES	1 TSP CANOLA OIL

Mix the ground meat with the garlic, vinegar, chili flakes and ginger in a bowl.

Heat oil in a skillet over a medium heat.

Add the beef to the pan and cook for 20-25 minutes or until cooked through.

Serve beef mixture with diced cucumber in each lettuce wrap and fold.

AROMATIC LAMB CURRY

SERVES 2　　PREP TIME: 10 MINUTES　　COOK TIME: 45 MINUTES

Fresh, zingy and hot all at the same time!

- 2 X LAMB STEAKS, SLICED INTO STRIPS
- 1 TBSP COCONUT OIL
- 1 GARLIC CLOVE, MINCED
- 1/2 STICK OF LEMON GRASS, VERY FINELY DICED
- 1/4 CUP OF HOMEMADE CHICKEN BROTH
- 1/4 CUP LOW FAT COCONUT MILK
- 1/2 TSP CURRY POWDER
- 1/2 ONION, CHOPPED
- 1 TBSP OF FRESH GINGER, GRATED
- 1/2 CUP OF TENDER-STEM OR SPROUTING BROCCOLI
- 1 STEM OF GREEN ONION, SLICED
- 1 CUPS COOKED BROWN RICE

Heat the coconut oil and garlic in a large pan over a medium to high heat for 2 minutes.

Add the lamb slices to the pan and brown each side for 2 minutes.

Once browned, remove lamb from the plan and place to one side.

Mix the ginger, curry powder, lemongrass and ¼ of the homemade chicken broth in a separate bowl.

Pour the broth mix, along with the broccoli into the pan.

Add the beef back into the pan along with the chopped onions.

Add the last of the broth and coconut milk over the lamb and simmer for 30-40 minutes or until piping hot and the beef is soft.

Serve piping hot with the green onion scattered over the top and rice on the side.

BEEF & PORK

APRICOT AND LAMB TAGINE

SERVES 2   PREP TIME: 10 MINUTES   COOK TIME: 1-1.5 HOURS

Aromatic and wonderful!

---

1 TBSP OF EXTRA VIRGIN OLIVE OIL	1 TSP TURMERIC
2 LEAN LAMB FILLETS, CUBED	1 TSP CURRY POWDER
1 ONION, DICED	1 TSP DRIED ROSEMARY
4 CUPS OF HOMEMADE CHICKEN STOCK	1 TSP OF CHOPPED PARSLEY
1 TSP CUMIN	1/2 CUP DRIED APRICOTS

Heat the olive oil in a large oven-proof pot over a medium high heat on the stove.

Add the lamb to the pot and cook for 5 minutes until browned.

Remove lamb and place to one side.

Add the chopped onion to the pot and saute for 5 minutes until starting to soften.

Sprinkle the cumin, turmeric and curry powder over the onions and continue to stir for 4-5 minutes.

Now add the lamb back into the pot with the chicken stock and rosemary.

Then cover the pot and leave to simmer on a low heat for 1-1.5 hours until the lamb is tender and fully cooked through.

Add the apricots 15 minutes before the end of the cooking time.

Plate up and serve with the chopped parsley to garnish.

Top tip: Once you've done step 1-5 you can complete the next steps in a slow cooker/dutch oven and leave on a medium heat overnight.

POULTRY MAIN DISHES

TOMATO & OLIVE CHICKEN FIESTA

SERVES 2   PREP TIME: 5 MINUTES   COOK TIME: 40 MINUTES

A taste of the Meditteranean!

- 2 FREE RANGE SKINLESS CHICKEN BREASTS
- 1 ONION, ROUGHLY CHOPPED
- 2 GARLIC CLOVES, CHOPPED
- 2 CANS CHOPPED TOMATOES
- 1 TBSP BALSAMIC VINEGAR
- 8 GREEN OLIVES, CHOPPED
- 2 CUPS HOMEMADE CHICKEN STOCK
- HANDFUL OF FRESH BASIL LEAVES
- A PINCH OF BLACK PEPPER

Preheat oven to 375°F/190 °C/Gas Mark 5.

Add the onion, garlic, chopped tomatoes, olives, chicken stock and balsamic vinegar to the pan with most of the basil leaves and cover.

Place in the oven for 35-40 minutes or until chicken is cooked throughout.

Plate up and serve with the remaining basil as a garnish.

CAJUN CHICKEN & PRAWN

SERVES 2   PREP TIME: 5 MINUTES   COOK TIME: 35 MINUTES

A very tasty recipe, inspired by Cajun cuisine.

- 2 FREE RANGE SKINLESS CHICKEN BREASTS, CHOPPED
- 1 ONION, CHOPPED
- 1 RED PEPPER, CHOPPED
- 2 GARLIC CLOVES, CRUSHED
- 10 FRESH OR FROZEN KING PRAWNS
- 1 TSP CAYENNE PEPPER
- 1 TSP CHILI POWDER
- 1 TSP PAPRIKA
- 1/4 TSP CHILI POWDER
- 1 TSP DRIED OREGANO
- 1 TSP DRIED THYME
- 1 CUP BROWN OR WHOLEGRAIN RICE
- 1 TBSP EXTRA VIRGIN OLIVE OIL
- 1 CAN CHOPPED TOMATOES
- 2 CUPS HOMEMADE CHICKEN STOCK

Mix the spices and herbs in a separate bowl to form your Cajun spice mix.

Grab a large pan and add the olive oil, heating on a medium heat.

Add the chicken and brown each side for around 4-5 minutes. Place to one side.

Add the onion to the pan and fry until soft.

Add the garlic, prawns, Cajun seasoning and red pepper to the pan and cook for around 5 minutes or until prawns become opaque.

Add the brown rice along with the chopped tomatoes, chicken and chicken stock to the pan.

Cover the pan and allow to simmer for around 25 minutes or until the rice is soft.

Serve and enjoy!

HEALTHY TURKEY GUMBO

SERVES 4   PREP TIME: 5 MINUTES   COOK TIME: 2 HOURS

An all-American staple that you can enjoy the anti-inflammatory way!

- 1 WHOLE TURKEY
- 1 ONION, QUARTERED
- A STALK OF CELERY, CHOPPED
- 3 CLOVES GARLIC, CHOPPED
- 1/2 CUP OKRA
- 1 CAN CHOPPED TOMATOES
- 1 TBSP EXTRA VIRGIN OLIVE OIL
- 1-2 BAY LEAVES
- BLACK PEPPER TO TASTE

Take the first four ingredients and add with 2 cups of water in a stockpot, heating on a high heat until boiling.

Lower the heat and simmer for 45-50 minutes or until turkey is cooked through.

Remove the turkey and strain the broth.

Grab a skillet and then heat the oil on a medium heat and brown the rest of the vegetables for 5-10 minutes.

Stir until tender and then add to the broth.

Add the tomatoes and turkey meat to the broth and stir.

Add the bay leaves and continue to cook for an hour or until sauce has thickened.

Season with black pepper and enjoy.

CHINESE ORANGE-SPICED DUCK BREASTS

SERVES 2   PREP TIME: 4 MINUTES   COOK TIME: 20 MINUTES

This citrus infused duck is bursting with flavor and easier to cook than you think!

- 1 TSP EXTRA VIRGIN OLIVE OIL FOR COOKING
- 2 DUCK BREASTS, SKIN REMOVED
- 1 WHITE ONION, SLICED
- 3 CLOVES GARLIC, MINCED
- 2 TSP GINGER, GRATED
- 1 TSP CINNAMON
- 1 TSP CLOVES
- 1 ORANGE – ZEST AND JUICE (RESERVE THE WEDGES)
- 2 BOK OR PAK CHOI PLANTS, LEAVES SEPARATED

Slice the duck breasts into strips and add to a dry hot pan, cooking for 5-7 minutes on each side or until cooked through to your liking.

Remove to one side.

Add olive oil to a clean pan and sauté the onions with the ginger, garlic and the rest of the spices for 1 minute.

Add the juice and zest of the orange and continue to sauté for 3-5 minutes.

Add the duck and bok choi and heat through until wilted and duck is piping hot.

Serve and garnish with the orange segments.

HARISSA SPICED CHICKEN TRAY-BAKE

SERVES 4   PREP TIME: 10 MINUTES   COOK TIME: 35 MINUTES

When time is limited but you don't want flavor to be! This should be a weeknight staple in any home!

---

4 FREE RANGE SKINLESS CHICKEN BREASTS, DICED

1/2 CUP OF LOW-FAT GREEK YOGURT

1 SMALL BUTTERNUT SQUASH, CHOPPED AND PEELED

2 RED ONIONS, CHOPPED

FOR THE HARISSA PASTE:

1 RED PEPPER, DICED

1 TSP DRIED RED CHILLI,
1 GARLIC CLOVE, MINCED

1 TSP CARAWAY SEEDS, CRUSHED
1 TSP GROUND CUMIN

1 TSP FRESH OR DRIED CORIANDER,

1 TBSP TOMATO PURÉE (NO ADDED SALT OR SUGAR)

1 TBSP EXTRA VIRGIN OLIVE OIL

Pre-heat oven to 375°F/190 °C/Gas Mark 5.

In a bowl, combine the ingredients for the harissa paste and then add 3 tbsp yogurt.

Coat the chicken breasts with the mixture, cover and leave to one side.

Scatter the chicken pieces, onions and chopped butternut squash with the harissa paste over a baking tray and place in the oven for 35 minutes or until the chicken is cooked right through.

Plate up and serve with the remaining yogurt.

Top tip: double up the harissa spices and save some for cooking later on – it tastes great on fish, chicken, turkey and even simple roast Mediterranean vegetables.

TERRIFIC TURKEY BURGERS

SERVES 2   PREP TIME: 5 MINUTES   COOK TIME: 35 MINUTES

Healthy turkey burgers - great if you've decided to cut out red meat.

- 8 OZ LEAN GROUND TURKEY MEAT
- 1 WHITE ONIONS, MINCED
- 1 CARROT, SHREDDED
- 2 CELERY STALKS, FINELY CHOPPED
- 1 RED BELL PEPPER, FINELY CHOPPED (OPTIONAL)
- 1 TBSP DILL
- 1 TSP CILANTRO
- 1 TSP DRY MUSTARD
- 2 TBSP OLIVE OIL
- PINCH OF BLACK PEPPER TO TASTE

Pre-heat oven to 390°F/200 °C/Gas Mark 6.

Add the vegetables in a bowl with the olive oil, pepper and herbs and then mix well.

Add in the meat and mix with wet hands to create two patties.

Place the patties on a lightly oiled baking tray and bake in the oven for 25-30 minutes or until meat is cooked through (flip half way).

Turn up the broiler and broil for the last 5 minutes for a golden and crispy edge.

Serve on a bed of your favorite salad.

Top tip: an egg helps the burger mixture stick together - try adding if you can eat eggs.

SUPER SESAME CHICKEN NOODLES

SERVES 2   PREP TIME: 10 MINUTES   COOK TIME: 20 MINUTES

Go ahead and mix things up with this tasty recipe.

---

2 FREE RANGE SKINLESS CHICKEN BREASTS, CHOPPED

1 CUP RICE/BUCKWHEAT NOODLES SUCH AS JAPANESE UDON

1 CARROT, CHOPPED

1/2 ORANGE, JUICED

1 TSP SESAME SEEDS

2 TSP COCONUT OIL

1 THUMB SIZED PIECE OF GINGER, MINCED

1/2 CUP SUGAR SNAP PEAS

Heat 1 tsp oil on a medium heat in a skillet.

Sauté the chopped chicken breast for about 10-15 minutes or until cooked through.

While cooking the chicken, place the noodles, carrots and peas in a pot of boiling water for about 5 minutes. Drain.

In a bowl, mix together the ginger, sesame seeds, 1 tsp oil and orange juice to make your dressing.

Once chicken is cooked and noodles are cooked and drained, add the chicken, noodles, carrots and peas to the dressing and toss.

Serve warm or chilled.

LEBANESE CHICKEN KEBABS AND HUMMUS

SERVES 4   PREP TIME: 10 MINUTES (MARINATE AS LONG AS POSSIBLE)
COOK TIME: 25 MINUTES

This is a spicy and hot chicken recipe inspired by Lebanese cuisine.

FOR THE CHICKEN:

1 CUP LEMON JUICE

8 GARLIC CLOVES, MINCED

1 TBSP THYME, FINELY CHOPPED

1 TBSP PAPRIKA

2 TSP GROUND CUMIN

1 TSP CAYENNE PEPPER

4 FREE RANGE SKINLESS CHICKEN BREASTS, CUBED

4 METAL KEBAB SKEWERS

LEMON WEDGES TO GARNISH

FOR THE HUMMUS:

1 CAN CHICKPEAS/ 1 CUP DRIED CHICKPEAS SOAKED OVERNIGHT

2 TBSP TAHINI PASTE

1 LEMON, JUICED

1 TSP TURMERIC

1 TSP BLACK PEPPER

2 TBSP OLIVE OIL

Whisk the lemon juice, garlic, thyme, paprika, cumin, and cayenne pepper in a bowl.

Skewer the chicken cubes using kebab sticks (metal).

Baste the chicken on each side with the marinade, covering for as long as possible in the fridge (the lemon juice will tenderize the meat and means it will be more suitable for the anti-inflammatory diet).

When ready to cook, preheat the oven to 400°F/200 °C/Gas Mark 6 and bake for 20-25 minutes or until chicken is thoroughly cooked through.

Prepare the hummus by adding the ingredients to a blender and whizzing up until smooth. If it is a little thick and chunky, add a little water to loosen the mix.

Serve the chicken kebabs, garnished with the lemon wedges and the hummus on the side.

ITALIAN CHICKEN & ZUCCHINI SPAGHETTI

SERVES 2   PREP TIME: 10 MINUTES   COOK TIME: 30 MINUTES

Fresh and simple, yet mouthwatering and amazing!

FOR THE CHICKEN:

- 2 FREE RANGE SKINLESS CHICKEN BREAST, SLICED
- 1 TBSP EXTRA VIRGIN OLIVE OIL
- JUICE OF 1/2 LEMON
- 1 CLOVE GARLIC, CRUSHED
- 1/2 TSP DRIED OREGANO
- PINCH OF BLACK PEPPER

FOR THE PASTA:

- 3 ZUCCHINIS
- 1 TSP EXTRA VIRGIN OLIVE OIL

Pre-heat oven to 400°F/200°C/Gas Mark 6.

Combine 1 tbsp olive oil, lemon juice, garlic, and oregano and coat the chicken slices.

Line a baking sheet with foil or parchment paper.

Layer the chicken strips and cook for 25-30 minutes or until cooked through.

Meanwhile, prepare your zucchini by slicing into thin spaghetti strips – use a mandolin or spiralyzer and leave in a colander to drain for 10 minutes.

When chicken is cooked, remove from the oven and place to one side.

Boil a pan of water on a medium heat and add a pinch of black pepper.

Add your zucchini spaghetti to the water and boil for one minute before immediately draining.

Plate and serve, layering half the chicken on top and drizzling with 1 tsp olive oil and a little black pepper. Enjoy!

GREEK FENNEL & OLIVE BAKED CHICKEN

SERVES 4   PREP TIME: 10 MINUTES   COOK TIME: 1 HOUR

A taste of the Aegean sea!

- 1 WHOLE FREE RANGE CHICKEN
- 1 TSP BLACK PEPPER
- 2 LEMONS, CUT INTO SLICES
- 3 CLOVES GARLIC, MINCED
- 1 TBSP OREGANO, CHOPPED
- 2 TBSP EXTRA VIRGIN OLIVE OIL
- 1 FENNEL BULB, SLICED
- 1/3 CUP PITTED BLACK OR KALAMATA OLIVES, HALVED
- 2 WHITE SWEET POTATOES, PEELED AND CUBED

Pre-heat oven to 375°F/190 °C/Gas Mark 5.

Pat the chicken dry with kitchen towel and place on a lined baking tray.

Use a sharp knife to slide underneath the skin and create a pocket. Sprinkle pepper underneath the skin.

Mix 1 tbsp olive oil, lemon zest and juice of the lemons with the garlic and oregano (save the lemon wedges).

Pour this into the pocket you created under the skin to marinate for as little or as much time as you have (don't worry if it drizzles out of the pocket).

Toss the fennel, sweet potato and olives, 1 tbsp oil and the lemon wedges in a separate bowl.

Scatter the fennel mix around the base of the chicken.

Bake for 1 hour or following package guidelines to ensure chicken is thoroughly cooked through. Remove the skin and cut into servings of the breasts, legs, thighs and any extra flaky meat you can cut away.

Serve immediately with an extra squeeze of lemon juice and some fresh thyme or oregano if desired!

ROSEMARY CHICKEN & SWEET POTATO STEW

SERVES 4   PREP TIME: 5 MINUTES   COOK TIME: 40 MINUTES

A tasty and wholesome low fat and low carb chicken recipe.

- 4 FREE RANGE SKINLESS CHICKEN THIGHS
- 1 WHITE ONION, CHOPPED
- 2 GARLIC CLOVES, SLICED
- 4 SWEET POTATOES, PEELED AND CUBED
- A PINCH OF BLACK PEPPER
- 1 TSP EXTRA VIRGIN OLIVE OIL
- 1 CAN OF CHOPPED TOMATOES
- 2 TBSP CHOPPED ROSEMARY LEAVES
- 2 TBSP BASIL LEAVES

Pre-heat oven to 375°F/190 °C/Gas Mark 5.

Heat oil in a pan on a medium heat and add the onion and garlic and cook for 5 minutes or until soft.

Pour in the chopped tomatoes, rosemary and pepper and cook for around 15 minutes until the mixture starts to thicken.

Place the chicken and sweet potato into a baking dish and pour over the sauce before transferring to the oven. Top up with a little water to ensure the chicken and potatoes are covered.

Bake for 20-25 minutes or until the chicken is cooked right through.

Check every now and then to ensure it doesn't dry up, adding a little water if necessary.

Sprinkle the basil on top to serve.

Top Tip: Double up to make in bulk and save the rest in a sealable container for 2-3 days. This also tastes amazing whizzed up in a blender as a soup!

NUTTY PESTO CHICKEN SUPREME

SERVES 2   PREP TIME: 10 MINUTES   COOK TIME: 30 MINUTES

Making your own pesto tastes so much more delightful and means you can control the ingredients going in – ideal for anti-inflammatory diets!

2 FREE RANGE SKINLESS CHICKEN OR TURKEY BREASTS	1 CUP CRUSHED MACADAMIAS/ ALMONDS/WALNUTS OR A COMBINATION
1 BUNCH OF FRESH BASIL	2 TBSP EXTRA VIRGIN OLIVE OIL
1/2 CUP RAW SPINACH	1/2 CUP LOW FAT HARD CHEESE (OPTIONAL)

Preheat oven to 350°f/170°c/Gas Mark 4.

Take the chicken breasts and use a meat pounder to 'thin' each breast into a 1cm thick escalope.

Reserve a handful of the nuts before adding the rest of the ingredients and a little black pepper to a blender or pestle and mortar and blend until smooth (you can leave this a little chunky for a rustic feel if you wish).

Add a little water if the pesto needs loosening.

Coat the chicken in the pesto.

Bake for at least 30 minutes in the oven, or until chicken is completely cooked through.

Top each chicken escalope with the remaining nuts and place under the broiler for 5 minutes for a crispy topping to complete.

MEDITTERANEAN CHICKEN

SERVES 2 / PREP TIME: 5 MINUTES / COOK TIME: 40 MINUTES

A taste of the Meditteranean!

- 2 FREE RANGE SKINLESS CHICKEN BREASTS
- 1 RED ONION, ROUGHLY CHOPPED
- 2 GARLIC CLOVES, CHOPPED
- 1 ZUCCHINI, CHOPPED
- 1 TBSP BALSAMIC VINEGAR
- 1 SWEET POTATO, PEELED AND CUBED
- 2 CUPS HOMEMADE CHICKEN STOCK
- 2 TBSP OREGANO
- A PINCH OF BLACK PEPPER

Preheat oven to 375°F/190 °C/Gas Mark 5.

Add the onion, garlic, zucchini, sweet potato, chicken stock, oregano and balsamic vinegar to the pan and cover.

Place in the oven for 35-40 minutes or until chicken is cooked throughout.

Plate up and serve hot.

CAJUN CHICKEN & CILANTRO QUINOA

SERVES 2   PREP TIME: 5 MINUTES   COOK TIME: 35 MINUTES

A very tasty recipe, inspired by Cajun cuisine.

- 2 FREE RANGE SKINLESS CHICKEN BREASTS, CHOPPED
- 1 ONION, CHOPPED
- 2 GARLIC CLOVES, CRUSHED
- 1 TSP CAYENNE PEPPER
- 1 TSP CHILI POWDER
- 1/4 TSP CHILI FLAKES
- 1 TSP DRIED OREGANO
- 1 TSP DRIED THYME
- 1 CUP QUINOA
- 1 TBSP CILANTRO, CHOPPED
- 1 TBSP EXTRA VIRGIN OLIVE OIL
- 2 CUPS HOMEMADE CHICKEN STOCK

Mix the spices and herbs in a separate bowl to form your Cajun spice mix (save the cilantro).

Grab a large pan and add the olive oil, heating on a medium heat.

Add the chicken and brown each side for around 4-5 minutes. Place to one side.

Add the onion to the pan and fry until soft.

Add the garlic, Cajun seasoning and chili flakes to the pan and cook for around 5 minutes.

Add the quinoa along with the chicken and chicken stock to the pan.

Cover the pan and allow to simmer for around 25 minutes or until the rice is soft. Serve and enjoy!

Top tip: multiply the quantities of the spices to make a Cajun spice mix that you can use again –just keep in a sealable jar or Tupperware somewhere dry!

TURKEY NOODLES

SERVES 2   PREP TIME: 10 MINUTES   COOK TIME: 20 MINUTES

The fresh vegetables taste delicious with the juice of the lime

---

- 2 SKINLESS TURKEY BREASTS, SLICED
- 1 CUP RICE/BUCKWHEAT NOODLES SUCH AS JAPANESE UDON
- 1/4 CUP BEANSPROUTS
- 1/2 LIME, ZEST & JUICE
- 1 TSP SESAME SEEDS
- 2 TSP COCONUT OIL
- 1 THUMB SIZED PIECE OF GINGER, MINCED
- 1/2 CUP SUGAR SNAP PEAS

Heat 1 tsp oil on a medium heat in a skillet.

Sauté the turkey breast for 10-15 minutes or until cooked through.

Add the beansprouts to the skillet for 5 minutes.

While cooking the chicken, place the noodles and sugar snap peas in a pot of boiling water for about 5 minutes. Drain.

In a bowl, mix together the ginger, sesame seeds, 1 tsp oil and lime juice to make your dressing.

Once turkey is cooked and noodles are cooked and drained, add the chicken, noodles, beansprouts and peas to the dressing and toss.

Sprinkle with a little lime zest.

Serve warm or chilled.

CHICKEN PESTO & AVOCADO SALAD

SERVES 2   PREP TIME: 10 MINUTES   COOK TIME: 30 MINUTES

Tasty homemade pesto and chicken breasts.

- 2 FREE RANGE SKINLESS CHICKEN OR TURKEY BREASTS
- 1 BUNCH OF FRESH BASIL
- 1/2 CUP RAW SPINACH
- 1 CUP CRUSHED MACADAMIAS
- 2 TBSP EXTRA VIRGIN OLIVE OIL
- 1/2 CUP LOW FAT HARD CHEESE (OPTIONAL)
- 1 AVOCADO
- 1/2 CUP ROMAINE LETTUCE LEAVES

Preheat oven to 350°f/170°c/Gas Mark 4.

Take the chicken breasts and use a meat pounder to 'thin' each breast into a 1cm thick escalope.

Reserve a handful of the nuts before adding the rest of the ingredients and a little black pepper to a blender or pestle and mortar and blend until smooth (you can leave this a little chunky for a rustic feel if you wish).

Add a little water if the pesto needs loosening.

Coat the chicken in the pesto.

Bake for at least 30 minutes in the oven, or until chicken is completely cooked through.

Top each chicken escalope with the remaining nuts and place under the broiler for 5 minutes for a crispy topping to complete.

Slice the chicken into strips.

Peel and slice your avocado and wash your lettuce leaves.

Serve the chicken strips and avocado on a bed of lettuce. Drizzle any leftover pesto over the salad if you wish!

SEAFOOD MAIN DISHES

GINGER & CHILI SEA BASS FILLETS

SERVES 2   PREP TIME: 5 MINUTES   COOK TIME: 10 MINUTES

Fresh and spicy, this Seabass dish is a must-try!

- 2 SEA BASS FILLETS
- 1 TSP BLACK PEPPER
- 1 TBSP EXTRA VIRGIN OLIVE OIL
- 1 TSP GINGER, PEELED AND CHOPPED
- 1 GARLIC CLOVE, THINLY SLICED
- 1 RED CHILI, DESEEDED AND THINLY SLICED
- 2 GREEN ONION STEMS, SLICED

Get a skillet and heat the oil on a medium to high heat.

Sprinkle black pepper over the Sea Bass and score the skin of the fish a few times with a sharp knife.

Add the sea bass fillet to the very hot pan with the skin side down.

Cook for 5 minutes and turn over.

Cook for a further 2 minutes.

Remove seabass from the pan and rest.

Add the chili, garlic and ginger and cook for approximately 2 minutes or until golden.

Remove from the heat and add the green onions.

Scatter the vegetables over your sea bass to serve.

Try with a steamed sweet potato or side salad.

SMOKED HADDOCK & PEA RISOTTO

SERVES 2   PREP TIME: 4 MINUTES   COOK TIME: 40 MINUTES

Risotto is amazing but most recipes call for risotto rice - use brown for an anti-inflammatory dish!

2 SMOKED HADDOCK FILLETS SKINLESS, BONELESS	1 CUP FRESH SPINACH LEAVES
1 TBSP EXTRA VIRGIN OLIVE OIL	1 CUP OF FROZEN PEAS
1 WHITE ONION, FINELY DICED	3 TBSP LOW FAT GREEK YOGURT (OPTIONAL)
2 CUPS BROWN RICE	A PINCH OF BLACK PEPPER
4 CUPS VEGETABLE STOCK	4 LEMON WEDGES
	1 CUP OF ARUGULA

Heat the oil in a large pan on a medium heat.

Sauté the chopped onion for 5 minutes until soft before adding in the rice and stirring for 1-2 minutes.

Add half of the stock and stir slowly.

Slowly add the rest of the stock whilst continuously stirring for up to 20-30 minutes (this is a bit of a workout!)

Stir in the spinach and peas to the risotto.

Place the fish on top of the rice, cover and steam for 10 minutes.

Use your fork to break up the fish fillets and stir into the rice with the yogurt.

Sprinkle with freshly ground pepper to serve and a squeeze of fresh lemon.

Garnish with the lemon wedges and serve with the arugula.

TASTY NUTTY TROUT

SERVES 2   PREP TIME: 5 MINUTES   COOK TIME: 15 MINUTES

This fish is so nutritious and the nuts add a lovely taste and texture!

---

2 TROUT FILLETS

1/2 CUP WHOLE WHEAT BREADCRUMBS

1 TBSP EXTRA VIRGIN OLIVE OIL

1/2 CUP FRESH PARSLEY, FINELY CHOPPED

ZEST AND JUICE OF 1 LEMON

1/2 CUP CHOPPED ALMONDS

Preheat the broiler on a high heat.

Lightly oil a baking tray.

Mix the breadcrumbs, parsley, lemon zest and juice and half of the nuts together in a shallow dish.

Lay the fillets skin side down onto the oiled baking tray and then flip over so that both sides of your fish are coated in the oil.

Now, dip the fillets into the nut mixture on both sides to coat.

Return to the baking tray.

Broil for 6-7 minutes on each side and serve with a side salad or vegetables of your choice.

PARSLEY & LEMON SPANISH SHRIMP

SERVES 2   PREP TIME: 10 MINUTES   COOK TIME: 20 MINUTES

This shrimp is influenced by Spanish paella dishes and is really easy to prepare!

- 2 CUPS WILD OR BASMATI RICE
- 4 CUPS OF WATER
- 12 WHOLE SHRIMP, PEELED, DEVEINED AND THE TAILS STILL INTACT
- 2 GARLIC CLOVES, CRUSHED
- 1 WHITE ONION, DICED
- 2 TBSP EXTRA VIRGIN OLIVE OIL
- 1/2 TSP RED PEPPER FLAKES
- 1 TBSP PARSLEY, CRUSHED
- 1 LEMON, JUICE AND ZEST
- 1 LEMON – CUT INTO QUARTERS

Add the rice and 4 cups of water to a saucepan and boil on a high heat.

Once boiling, lower the heat, cover and simmer for 15 minutes.

Meanwhile heat the oil in a skillet on a medium heat and then sauté the onion, garlic and red pepper flakes for 5 minutes until softened and then add the shrimp.

Sauté for 5-8 minutes or until shrimp is opaque

Drain the rice and return to the heat for a further 3 minutes with the lid on.

Add the rice to the shrimps.

Add in the parsley, zest and juice of 1 lemon and mix well.

Serve in a wide paella dish if possible or a large serving dish – scatter the lemon wedges around the edge and sprinkle with a little more fresh parsley.

Season with black pepper to taste.

NUT-CRUST TILAPIA WITH KALE

SERVES 2   PREP TIME: 5 MINUTES   COOK TIME: 15 MINUTES

The crunchy topping on this fish makes it stand out from the crowd and the kale is rich in vitamins and iron.

---

2 TSP EXTRA VIRGIN OLIVE OIL

2 TBSP LOW FAT HARD CHEESE CHEESE, GRATED

1/2 CUP ROASTED AND GROUND BRAZIL NUTS/HAZELNUTS/ANY OTHER HARD NUT

1/2 CUP 100% WHOLEGRAIN BREAD CRUMBS

2 TILAPIA FILLETS, SKINLESS

2 TSP WHOLE GRAIN MUSTARD

1 HEAD OF KALE, CHOPPED

1 TBSP SESAME SEEDS, LIGHTLY TOASTED

1 CLOVE OF GARLIC, MASHED

Preheat oven to 350°f/170°c/Gas Mark 4.

Lightly oil a baking sheet with 1 tsp extra virgin olive oil.

Mix in the nuts, breadcrumbs, and cheese in a separate bowl.

Spread a thin layer of the mustard over the fish and then dip into the breadcrumb mixture.

Transfer to baking dish.

Bake for 12 minutes or until cooked through.

Meanwhile, heat 1 tsp oil in a skillet on a medium heat and sauté the garlic for 30 seconds, adding in the kale for a further 5 minutes.

Mix in the sesame seeds.

Serve the fish at once with the kale on the side.

WASABI SALMON BURGERS

SERVES 4   PREP TIME: 5 MINUTES   COOK TIME: 10 MINUTES

A fish burger with a punch – a little Japanese US fusion!

- 1/2 TSP HONEY
- 2 TBSP REDUCED-SALT SOY SAUCE
- 1 TSP WASABI POWDER
- 1 BEATEN FREE RANGE EGG
- 2 CANS OF WILD SALMON, DRAINED
- 2 SCALLIONS, CHOPPED
- 2 TBSP COCONUT OIL
- 1 TBSP FRESH GINGER, MINCED

Combine the salmon, egg, ginger, scallions and 1 tbsp oil in a bowl, mixing well with your hands to form 4 patties.

In a separate bowl, add the wasabi powder and soy sauce with the honey and whisk until blended.

Heat 1 tbsp oil over a medium heat in a skillet and cook the patties for 4 minutes each side until firm and browned.

Glaze the top of each patty with the wasabi mixture and cook for another 15 seconds before you serve.

Serve with your favorite side salad or vegetables for a healthy treat.

SALMON & LIME WITH ARUGULA

SERVES 2   PREP TIME: 2 MINUTES   COOK TIME: 10 MINUTES

Rich in omega-3 and iron, this is super brain food!

FOR THE FISH:

2 SKINLESS SALMON FILLETS

1 TBSP EXTRA VIRGIN OLIVE OIL

1/2 FRESH LIME, JUICED

A PINCH OF BLACK PEPPER TO TASTE

FOR THE SALAD:

4 CUPS BABY ARUGULA LEAVES

1 CUP GRAPES OR CHERRY TOMATOES, CUT INTO HALVES

1/2 CUP SLIVERED RED ONION

1 TBSP OLIVE OIL

1 TBSP BALSAMIC VINEGAR

In a bowl, coat the salmon with the olive oil, lime juice and pepper (if you can, leave for at least 15 minutes up to an hour but don't worry if not).

Heat the oil in a skillet over a medium heat and cook the salmon skin-side for about 4-5 minutes each side or until completely cooked through.

Add the arugula, onion and tomatoes with oil and vinegar to a separate bowl and toss.

Serve the fish on the bed of salad.

SPICY COD BROTH

SERVES 2   PREP TIME: 10 MINUTES   COOK TIME: 20 MINUTES

An aromatic and spicy bowl of goodness.

---

2 BLACK COD FILLETS	3 HEADS OF BOK CHOY
A PINCH OF BLACK PEPPER	1 CARROT, SLICED
1 TSP REDUCED SODIUM SOY SAUCE	1 TBSP GINGER, MINCED
2 CUPS HOMEMADE CHICKEN BROTH (USE VEGETABLE IF YOU'VE GIVEN UP MEAT)	2 CUPS OF UDON NOODLES
	1 GREEN ONION, THINLY SLICED
1 TSP COCONUT OIL	2 TSP CILANTRO, FINELY CHOPPED
1 TSP FIVE-SPICE POWDER	1 TSP SESAME SEEDS
1 TBSP OLIVE OIL	

Rub the fish with pepper.

In a bowl, combine pepper, soy sauce, 1 cup chicken broth, coconut oil and spice blend. Mix together and place to one side.

In a large saucepan, heat the oil on a medium heat and cook the bok choy, ginger and carrot for about 2 minutes until the bok choy is green.

Add the rest of the reserved chicken stock and heat through.

Add the udon noodles and stir, bringing to a simmer.

Add the green onion and the fish and cook for 10-15 minutes until fish is tender.

Add the fish, noodles and vegetables into serving bowls and pour the broth over the top.

Garnish with the cilantro and sesame seeds and serve with chopsticks for real authenticity!

Top tip: This works with most types of white fish or even salmon so switch things up according to what's sustainable at the time of cooking!

BAKED GARLIC & LEMON HALIBUT

SERVES 2   PREP TIME: 5 MINUTES   COOK TIME: 15 MINUTES

Garlic is renowned for its anti-inflammatory properties and tastes delicious with this meaty fish.

- 2 HALIBUT FILLETS
- A PINCH OF BLACK PEPPER
- 2 GARLIC CLOVES, PRESSED
- 2 TBSP OLIVE OIL
- 4 LEMON WEDGES TO GARNISH

Preheat oven to 400°f/190°c/Gas Mark 5.

Season the fish with the pepper and add to a parchment paper-lined baking dish.

Scatter the garlic cloves (no need to peel) around the fish and drizzle with the oil.

Squeeze the lemon juice over the fish.

Bake for approximately 15 minutes until the fish is firm and well cooked.

Serve and pour over the juices for a delicious garlic feast.

Top tip: serve this with your preference of vegetable, salad or even sweet potato depending on your dietary requirements.

FRESH TUNA STEAK & FENNEL SALAD

SERVES 2   PREP TIME: 5 MINUTES   COOK TIME: 25 MINUTES

The aniseed taste of the fennel blends so well with the delicate peas and the meaty taste of the tuna.

2 TUNA STEAKS, EACH 1 INCH THICK	1 GARLIC CLOVE, CRUSHED
2 TBSP OLIVE OIL,	1 TSP CRUSHED FENNEL SEEDS
1 TBSP OLIVE OIL FOR BRUSHING	1 FENNEL BULB, TRIMMED AND SLICED
1 TSP CRUSHED BLACK PEPPERCORNS	1/2 CUP WATER
	1 LEMON, JUICED

Coat the fish with oil and then season with peppercorns and fennel seeds.

Heat the oil on a medium heat and sauté the fennel bulb slices for 5 minutes or until light brown, stir in the garlic and cook for another minute.

Add the water to the pan and cook for 10 minutes until fennel is tender.

Stir in the lemon juice and lower heat to a simmer.

Meanwhile, heat another skillet and sauté the tuna steaks for about 2-3 minutes each side for medium-rare. (Add 1 minute each side for medium and 2 minutes each side for medium well).

Serve the fennel mix with the tuna steaks on top and garnish with the fresh parsley.

SESAME MAHI-MAHI & FRUIT SALSA

SERVES 2   PREP TIME: 5 MINUTES   COOK TIME: 20 MINUTES

This fun tropical dish combines a great-tasting fish with a tangy salsa.

FOR THE SALSA:

1 CUP FRESH PINEAPPLE, PEELED AND CUBED

1/2 RED CHILI, FINELY CHOPPED

1 LIME, JUICED

2 TSP CILANTRO, CHOPPED

1 ONION, FINELY CHOPPED

FOR THE FISH:

2 MAHI MAHI FILLETS

2 TSP COCONUT OIL

2 TBSP SESAME SEEDS

Get a bowl and mix all of the ingredients for the salsa.

Drizzle 1 tbsp coconut oil on the fillets and coat each side with the sesame seeds.

Heat 1 tbsp oil over a medium heat and then sauté the fillets for about 8 minutes each side or until the flesh flakes away.

Serve with the salsa on the side.

SMOKED SALMON HASH BROWNS

SERVES 2   PREP TIME: 5 MINUTES   COOK TIME: 35 MINUTES

A yummy filling and healthy fish dish.

- 1 LARGE SWEET POTATO, PEELED AND CUBED
- 3 TBSP EXTRA VIRGIN OLIVE OIL
- 1 LEEK, CHOPPED
- 4 TSP DILL, CHOPPED
- 1 TBSP GRATED ORANGE PEEL
- 1 PACK SMOKED SALMON, SLICED
- 1 1/3 CUP LOW FAT GREEK YOGURT (OPTIONAL)

Preheat oven to 325°f/150°c/Gas Mark 3.

Lightly grease 2 ramekins or circular baking dishes with a little olive oil.

Heat the rest of the oil in a skillet over medium heat, and sauté the leeks and the potatoes for 5 minutes.

Lower the heat and cook for another 10 minutes until tender.

Transfer the potatoes and leeks to a separate bowl and crush with a fork to form a mash (alternatively use a potato masher).

Add the dill, orange peel and the salmon and mix well.

Fill the ramekins with half the mixture each, patting to compact.

Bake for 15 minutes and remove.

Serve hash in the ramekin, season and top with a dollop of Greek yogurt (optional).

SCRUMPTIOUS SCALLOPS WITH CILANTRO AND LIME

SERVES 2   PREP TIME: 5 MINUTES   COOK TIME: 5 MINUTES

Scallops are a delicacy and if you feel like pushing the boat out, a great tasty change from the norm!

---

8 QUEEN OR KING SCALLOPS (ROW ON)	1/2 LIME JUICE
1 TBSP EXTRA SESAME OIL	2 TBSP OF CHOPPED CILANTRO
2 LARGE GARLIC CLOVES, FINELY CHOPPED	A PINCH OF BLACK PEPPER
1 RED CHILI, FINELY CHOPPED	

Heat oil in a skillet on a medium to high heat and fry scallops for about 1 minute each side until lightly golden.

Add the chopped chili and garlic cloves to the pan and squeeze the lime juice over the scallops. Saute for 2-3 minutes.

Remove the scallops and sprinkle the cilantro and black pepper over the top to serve.

GLUTEN-FREE COCONUT SHRIMP BITES

SERVES 2   PREP TIME: 10 MINUTES   COOK TIME: 15 MINUTES

A healthy lightly battered shrimp dish.

---

2 CUPS SHRIMP, PEELED AND DEVEINED

1/4 CUP COCONUT FLOUR

1/2 TSP CAYENNE PEPPER

1 TSP GARLIC POWDER

2 BEATEN FREE RANGE EGGS

1/2 CUP SHREDDED COCONUT

1/4 CUP ALMOND FLOUR

A PINCH OF BLACK PEPPER TO TASTE

1 CUP ARUGULA OR WATERCRESS

Preheat oven to 400°f/200°c/Gas Mark 6.

Line a baking sheet with parchment paper.

Mix the coconut flour, cayenne pepper, and garlic powder in a bowl.

In a separate bowl, whisk the eggs.

In a third bowl, add the shredded coconut, almond flour and pepper.

Dip the shrimp into each dish in consecutive order, and then place on the baking sheet and bake for 10-15 minutes or until cooked through.

Serve piping hot and straight from the oven with a side salad of arugula or watercress.

CITRUS & HERB SARDINES

SERVES 2   PREP TIME: 5 MINUTES   COOK TIME: 15 MINUTES

Sardines are a great source of protein as well as omega 3's – they're recommended to eat between 2-6 times a week on the anti-inflammatory diet.

10 SARDINES, SCALED AND CLEANED (8 IF LARGE)	3 TBSP OLIVE OIL
ZEST OF 2 WHOLE LEMONS	1 CAN OF CHOPPED TOMATOES (OPTIONAL)
HANDFUL OF FLAT-LEAF PARSLEY, CHOPPED	1/2 CAN CHICKPEAS OR BUTTERBEANS, DRAINED AND RINSED
2 GARLIC CLOVES, FINELY CHOPPED	8 CHERRY TOMATOES, HALVED (OPTIONAL)
1/2 CUP BLACK OLIVES (PITTED AND HALVED)	A PINCH OF BLACK PEPPER

In a bowl add the lemon zest to the chopped parsley (save a pinch for garnishing) and half of the chopped garlic, ready for later.

Put a very large skillet on the hob and heat on high.

Now add the oil and once very hot, lay the sardines flat on the pan.

Saute for 3 minutes until golden underneath and turn over to fry for another 3 minutes. Place onto a plate to rest.

Sauté the remaining garlic (add another splash of oil if you need to) for 1 min until softened. Pour in the tin of chopped tomatoes, mix and let simmer for 4-5 minutes.

If you're avoiding tomatoes just avoid this step and go straight to chickpeas.

Tip in the chickpeas or butter beans and fresh tomatoes and stir until heated through.

Here's when you add the sardines into the lemon and parsley dressing prepared earlier and add to the pan, cooking for a further 3-4 minutes.

Once heated through, serve with a pinch of parsley and remaining lemon zest to garnish.

SPICY SHARK STEAKS

SERVES 2   PREP TIME: 35 MINUTES   COOK TIME: 40 MINUTES

A taste of the exotic! You can use tuna or monkfish in place of shark.

- 2 SHARK STEAKS, SKINLESS
- 2 TBSP ONION POWDER
- 2 TSP CHILI POWDER
- 1 GARLIC CLOVE, MINCED
- 1/4 CUP WORCESTERSHIRE SAUCE
- 1 TBSP GROUND BLACK PEPPER
- 2 TBSP THYME, CHOPPED

In a bowl, mix all of the seasonings and spices to form a paste before setting aside.

Spread a thin layer of paste on both sides of the fish, cover and chill for 30 minutes (If possible).

Preheat oven to 325°f/150°c/Gas Mark 3.

Bake the fish in parchment paper for 30-40 minutes, until well cooked.

Serve on a bed of quinoa or wholegrain couscous and your favorite salad.

SEABASS WITH PESTO MASH

SERVES 2   PREP TIME: 5 MINUTES   COOK TIME: 15 MINUTES

Great!

2X 3 OZ SEA BASS FILLETS	FOR THE PESTO:
1 TSP BLACK PEPPER	1/2 CUP FRESH BASIL
1 TBSP EXTRA VIRGIN OLIVE OIL	1/2 CUP FRESH SPINACH
FOR THE MASH:	1 TSP BLACK PEPPER
2 TURNIPS, PEELED AND CUBED	1/4 CUP EXTRA VIRGIN OLIVE OIL
	1 GARLIC CLOVE, MINCED
	1 LEMON, JUICED

Soak all your vegetables in warm water.

Prepare the pesto by blending all the ingredients for the pesto in a food processor or grinding with a pestle and mortar. Place to one side.

Boil a pan of water on a high heat and add the turnips.

Allow to boil for 20-25 minutes or until very soft.

Drain and use a potato masher to mash the turnips.

Fold the pesto through the mash.

Now grab a skillet and heat the oil over a medium to high heat.

Sprinkle black pepper over the sea bass fillet and score the skin of the fish a few times with a sharp knife.

Add the sea bass fillet to the very hot pan with the skin side down.

Cook for 7-8 minutes and turn over (this will allow the skin to turn crispy and golden).

Cook for a further 3-4 minutes or until cooked through.

Remove fillets from the skillet and allow to rest.

PARSLEY, LEMON & FENNEL TROUT

SERVES 2 / PREP TIME: 5 MINUTES / COOK TIME: 15 MINUTES

Fresh and delightful!

---

2 TROUT FILLETS

1/2 CUP WHOLE WHEAT GLUTEN-FREE BREADCRUMBS

1 TBSP EXTRA VIRGIN OLIVE OIL

1/2 CUP FRESH PARSLEY, FINELY CHOPPED

ZEST AND JUICE OF 1 LEMON

1 FENNEL BULB, SLICED

Preheat the broiler on a high heat.

Lightly oil a baking tray.

Mix the breadcrumbs, parsley, lemon zest and juice together in a shallow dish.

Lay the fillets skin side down onto the oiled baking tray and then flip over so that both sides of your fish are coated in the oil.

Now, dip the fillets into the breadcrumb mixture on both sides to coat.

Return to the baking tray.

Scatter the fennel slices around the fish.

Broil for 6-7 minutes on each side or until fish is thoroughly cooked through.

Serve with a side salad or vegetables of your choice.

SCALLOPS WITH CAULIFLOWER & APPLE

SERVES 2   PREP TIME: 5 MINUTES   COOK TIME: 10 MINUTES

What a treat!

---

6 QUEEN OR KING SCALLOPS (ROW ON)

1 TBSP COCONUT OIL

1/4 CAULIFLOWER

1/4 APPLE

A PINCH OF BLACK PEPPER

Wash the cauliflower and remove any leaves. Use a sharp knife to cut very thin slices of cauliflower.

Peel and remove core from the apple. Use a sharp knife to cut into 1/2cm thick cubes.

Add oil to a pan over a medium heat and add the apple pieces. Leave to cook and then stir once for 4-5 minutes.

Now add the cauliflower slices and cook for 3-4 minutes.

Remove apple and cauliflower from pan and add a little extra oil.

Saute scallops for about 1 minute each side until lightly golden.

Plate up the cauliflower slices and apple pieces and place the scallops on top before seasoning with black pepper to taste.

LEMON & PARSLEY MACKEREL

SERVES 2   PREP TIME: 5 MINUTES   COOK TIME: 15 MINUTES

Oily fish are recommended on the anti-inflammatory diet and taste amazing.

- 8 MACKEREL FILLETS, SCALED AND CLEANED
- ZEST OF 2 WHOLE LEMONS
- 1/2 CUP FLAT-LEAF PARSLEY, CHOPPED
- 2 GARLIC CLOVES, FINELY CHOPPED
- 1 LEMON, ZEST AND JUICE
- 3 TBSP OLIVE OIL
- 1/2 CAN CHICKPEAS OR BUTTERBEANS, DRAINED AND RINSED
- A PINCH OF BLACK PEPPER

In a bowl add the lemon juice to the chopped parsley (save a pinch for garnishing) and half of the chopped garlic, ready for later.

Put a very large skillet on the hob and heat on high.

Now add the oil and once very hot, lay the mackerel flat on the pan.

Sauté for 3 minutes until golden underneath and turn over for another 3 minutes.

Place onto a plate to rest.

Sauté the remaining garlic (add another splash of oil if you need to) for 1 min until softened.

Tip in the chickpeas or butter beans and stir until heated through.

Add the lemon and parsley dressing you prepared earlier to the pan, cooking for a further 3-4 minutes.

Once heated through, serve with a pinch of parsley and remaining lemon zest to garnish.

CURRIED MONKFISH

SERVES 2   PREP TIME: 35 MINUTES   COOK TIME: 40 MINUTES

A taste of the exotic!

---

2 MONKFISH STEAKS, SKINLESS

1 TSP TURMERIC

1 TSP CHILI POWDER

1 GARLIC CLOVE, MINCED

In a bowl, mix all of the seasoning's and spices to form a paste before setting aside.

Spread a thin layer of paste on both sides of the fish, cover and chill for 30 minutes (if possible).

Preheat oven to 325°f/150°c/Gas Mark 3.

Bake the fish, onions and garlic in parchment paper for 30-40 minutes, until thoroughly cooked through.

Serve with your choice of quinoa or salad and enjoy.

VEGETARIAN MAIN DISHES

LIME & SATAY TOFU WITH SUGARSNAPS

SERVES 2   PREP TIME: 5 MINUTES   COOK TIME: 15 MINUTES

Packed with protein and peanuty goodness.

- 1 PACK OF DRAINED, PRESSED AND CUBED TOFU
- 3 TBSP COCONUT OIL
- A PINCH OF BLACK PEPPER TO TASTE
- 1 CUP UDON NOODLES/BROWN RICE, COOKED
- 1 CUP OF SUGARSNAP PEAS

FOR THE SAUCE:
- 3 TBSP SOYBEAN MILK
- 1 TBSP WHOLE ALMOND BUTTER
- 2 TBSP REDUCED SODIUM OYSTER SAUCE
- 1 TBSP GARLIC POWDER
- 1 TSP CHILI FLAKES
- 1 TSP TOMATO PUREE (NO ADDED SUGAR OR SALT)
- 1 TSP LIME JUICE

Heat the oil on a high heat and then sauté the tofu until brown on each side.

Place onto paper towels to soak excess moisture and place to one side.

Heat the milk in a pan over a medium heat until starting to bubble and then add the peanut butter and the rest of the ingredients for the sauce, stirring continuously for 5 minutes until smooth and hot.

Add the tofu to the sauce, cooking for 4-5 minutes until heated through.

Meanwhile, steam or boil your sugar snap peas for 3-4 minutes.

Serve all ingredients piping hot with your choice of cooked udon noodles or brown rice.

LATINO BLACK BEAN STEW

SERVES 4   PREP TIME: 5 MINUTES   COOK TIME: 20 MINUTES

If you're craving the distinct taste of an authentic Mexican meal, this recipe is without the usual grease that comes hand in hand with the takeaway version!

- 1 CUP OF FRESHLY BROWN RICE
- 1 CUP OF FRESHLY QUINOA
- 1/2 CUP OF BLACK OLIVES, HALVED
- 1/2 CUP BLACK BEANS
- 1 AVOCADO, SLICED
- 2 TBSP OF PLAIN NON-FAT GREEK YOGURT
- 1 BEEF TOMATO, FINELY CHOPPED (OPTIONAL)
- 1/2 RED ONION, FINELY CHOPPED
- 1 LIME, JUICED
- 1 LIME, CUT INTO WEDGES
- 1 TBSP FRESH CILANTRO, FINELY CHOPPED

Heat a pan of water on a high heat and add brown rice, allowing to cook for 15 minutes.

Meanwhile, heat a separate pan of water on a high heat and add quinoa, allowing to cook for 15 minutes.

Add the black beans to the pan of rice to cook along with the rice.

Check most of the water in each pan has been absorbed, drain and cover on the heat for 2 minutes. Turn off heat.

Grab a large serving bowl and mix rice, quinoa, beans, olives, red onion, tomato and lime juice together.

In a separate bowl, crush the avocado into the yogurt with a fork and squeeze any remaining lime juice into the dip.

Enjoy your authentic Mexican meal, topped with cilantro, the avocado dip, and the lime wedges to serve.

Top tip: cook up rice and quionoa in batches and keep sealed in fridge so that you can make your favorite dishes quickly.

ZUCCHINI & PEPPER LASAGNA

SERVES 1 PREP TIME: 10 MINUTES COOK TIME: 1 HOUR

Very low in fat and vegan, this is quick and easy to prepare, using only a few ingredients; it's delicious and very filling too!

- 1/2 PACK OF SOFT TOFU
- 1/2 PACK OF FIRM TOFU
- WHOLEGRAIN LASAGNA SHEETS (1/2 BOX)
- 1 CUP BABY SPINACH
- 1 CUP OF ALMOND MILK
- 1/4 TSP OF GARLIC POWDER
- JUICE OF 1/2 A LEMON
- 1 1/2 TBSP OF FRESH BASIL, CHOPPED
- 1 CAN OF CHOPPED TOMATOES
- A PINCH OF BLACK PEPPER TO TASTE
- 1 ZUCCHINI, DICED
- 1 RED PEPPER, DICED (OPTIONAL)

Preheat oven to 325°F/170 °C/Gas Mark 3.

In a blender, process the soft and firm tofu, garlic powder, almond milk, basil, lemon juice and pepper until smooth.

Toss in the spinach and zucchini for the last 30 seconds.

Put about 1/3 of the chopped tomatoes at the bottom of an oven dish.

Top the sauce with 1/3 of the lasagna sheets and then 1/3 of the spinach/tofu mixture.

Repeat the layers finishing with the chopped tomatoes on top.

Cook for around 1 hour or until the pasta sheets are soft.

Serve with a lovely side salad and enjoy.

TOASTED CUMIN CRUNCH

SERVES 1   PREP TIME: 5 MINUTES   COOK TIME: 10 MINUTES

Cumin seeds are renowned for their anti-inflammatory properties and taste amazing with most salads and vegetables.

- 1 TBSP GROUND CUMIN SEEDS (USE A PESTLE AND MORTAR OR BLENDER)
- 2 TBSP EXTRA VIRGIN OLIVE OIL
- 1 TSP CRACKED BLACK PEPPERCORNS
- 1/2 TSP CUMIN SEEDS (WHOLE)
- 1 TSP CILANTRO, FINELY CHOPPED
- 1/2 JALAPENO, FINELY CHOPPED
- 2 CUPS OF GREEN CABBAGE, SLICED
- 2 CUPS OF CARROTS, GRATED
- 3 TBSP LIME JUICE

Get a large saucepan, and then heat the oil over a medium heat.

Cook the peppercorns, cilantro and the whole cumin seeds for about a minute until browned.

Add in the jalapeno and then cook for another 45 seconds until tender.

Add in then the carrots and the cabbage, cooking for about 5 minutes or until the cabbage starts to soften.

Add in the crushed cumin seeds and cook for 30 seconds before taking off the heat and then stirring in the lime juice and the cilantro.

Serve warm.

SPICY VEGETABLE BURGERS

SERVES 2   PREP TIME: 2 MINUTES   COOK TIME: 15 MINUTES

You needn't miss out on a sneaky treat just because you're vegetarian – try this delicious recipe and you'll be amazed.

EXTRA FIRM TEMPAH (1 PACK)

2 TBSP COCONUT OIL

1 TSP OF RED CHILI FLAKES

1 RED PEPPER, DICED (OPTIONAL)

1/2 RED ONION, DICED

1/2 CUP BABY SPINACH

1 TBSP OLIVE OIL

2 100% WHOLEGRAIN BUN (OPTIONAL)

1/2 CUP ARUGULA

Heat the broiler on a medium high heat.

Marinate the tempah in 1tbsp coconut oil and red chilli flakes.

Heat a 1 tbsp coconut oil in a skillet on a medium heat.

Sauté the onion in the skillet for 6-7 minutes or until caramelized.

Stir in the pepper and baby spinach for a further 3-4 minutes.

Broil the tempah for around 4 minutes on each side.

Lay down the tempah in the buns and then add the caramelized onion, spinach and diced peppers.

Serve immediately while hot with a side of arugla.

SUN DRIED TOMATO & NUT PASTA

SERVES 2   PREP TIME: 5 MINUTES   COOK TIME: 20 MINUTES

A delicious pasta dish.

- 1 CUP 100% WHOLEGRAIN PASTA
- 1 CLOVE OF GARLIC, MINCED
- 1/4 CUP OF WALNUTS, COARSELY CHOPPED
- 1/2 CUP SUN-DRIED TOMATOES, DRAINED & CHOPPED (OPTIONAL)
- 2 TBSP OF EXTRA VIRGIN OLIVE OIL
- 1 BUNCH FRESH BASIL, CHOPPED
- 100G OF LOW-FAT MOZZARELLA CHEESE
- PINCH OF BLACK PEPPER

Boil a large saucepan of water on a high heat.

Add the pasta and cook following directions on the package.

While the pasta is cooking, prepare the sauce:

Put minced garlic in a bowl.

Add sun-dried tomatoes, walnuts, basil, mozzarella and oil.

Once the pasta is cooked, drain and add to the sauce.

Toss through until the pasta is well coated.

Transfer onto a serving plate and sprinkle with a little black pepper.

Top tip: If you're avoiding wheat completely, prepare this dish with spiralyzed zucchini or carrots. Just cook in boiling water for 1-2 minutes and serve as you would pasta!

SPAGHETTI SQUASH & MARINATED TEMPAH

SERVES 2   PREP TIME: 15 MINUTES   COOK TIME: 50 MINUTES

Yummy!

- 1 PACK OF TEMPEH, DRAINED AND CUBED
- 1 SPAGHETTI SQUASH OR PUMPKIN, HALVED AND DESEEDED
- 3 TBSP OF TAMARI OR REDUCED SODIUM SOY SAUCE
- 1 CAN OF CHOPPED TOMATOES
- 1 TBSP OF EXTRA VIRGIN OLIVE OIL
- 2 CLOVES OF GARLIC, CHOPPED FINELY
- 1 CUP SMALL BROCCOLI FLORETS
- 1/2 CUP OF BABY SPINACH

Pre-heat the oven to 375°F/190 °C/Gas Mark 5. Get a medium-sized bowl and toss together the tamari, tempeh, garlic.

Marinate for as long as you can and up to overnight if possible.

Grab a large baking dish and arrange the squash halves with the cut side down and pour half a cup of water into the dish.

Bake for around 45 minutes or until tender and remove the dish from the oven. Turn the squash over and allow to slightly cool.

Get a large skillet and heat oil over a medium heat.

Add tempeh and cook for 7 to 8 minutes until golden brown, occasionally stirring.

Remove the tempeh and keep warm on a plate.

In a medium-sized pot, heat chopped tomatoes at medium heat, and then add the broccoli and allow to cook until tender (around 5 minutes.) Stir the spinach in and remove from heat.

Use a fork to scrape off spaghetti squash strands onto a platter. Spoon broccoli and hot chopped tomatoes over the dish.

Top with the tempeh to serve.

RUSTIC GARLIC AND CHIVE QUINOA

SERVES 2   PREP TIME: 5 MINUTES   COOK TIME: 30 MINUTES

A light and simple dish which can be experimented with by adding different flavors and vegetables.

1/2 CUP OF KIDNEY BEANS	3 GREEN ONION STALKS, DICED
1/2 CUP OF UNCOOKED QUINOA	4 CLOVES OF GARLIC, MINCED
2 CUPS OF VEGETABLE BROTH (LOW SALT)	1/4 TSP OF BLACK PEPPER
	1 TBSP EXTRA VIRGIN OLIVE OIL
1/2 WHITE ONION, DICED	

In a large pan, sautee garlic and onion in olive oil over a medium heat until the onions soften.

Lower the heat and add the quinoa, kidney beans and vegetable broth.

Cover the pan and simmer for around 15 to 20 minutes or until quinoa is soft and liquid is absorbed.

Serve with the diced green onion scattered over the quinoa and a little black pepper to taste.

PORTABELLA MUSHROOM CUPS

SERVES 4 PREP TIME: 5 MINUTES COOK TIME: 10 MINS

This is a unique and healthy entree recipe for vegetarians in need of a high-fiber meal.

- 4 LARGE PORTABELLA MUSHROOMS
- 1/2 CUP OF COOKED WILD RICE/BROWN RICE/QUINOA
- 1 RED BELL PEPPER, CHOPPED (OPTIONAL)
- 1 BEEF TOMATO, CHOPPED (OPTIONAL)
- 1/2 CUCUMBER, CHOPPED
- 1 GREEN ONION, SLICED
- 4 TSP OF EXTRA VIRGIN OLIVE OIL
- 1 TBSP OF DIJON MUSTARD
- 1 TBSP OF WHITE WINE VINEGAR
- PINCH OF BLACK PEPPER

Preheat the broiler to a medium high heat.

Combine the cooked quinoa, bell pepper, cucumber, green onion, mustard and white wine vinegar in a separate bowl.

Place the portabella mushrooms on a baking sheet and lightly brush with olive oil.

Stack the mushroom caps with the quinoa mixture.

Place under the broiler for 10 minutes, then serve immediately with black pepper to taste.

INDIAN BROCCOLI RABE & CAULIFLOWER

SERVES 4   PREP TIME: 5 MINUTES   COOK TIME: 25 MINUTES

This is a spicy, tasty vegetarian Indian dish.

- 1⁄2 BUNCH BROCCOLI RABE (RAPINI)
- 1/2 CAULIFLOWER, FLORETS
- 1 ONION, DICED
- 1 THUMB SIZED PIECE OF GINGER, MINCED
- 4 GARLIC CLOVES, MINCED
- 1 TSP BLACK MUSTARD SEEDS
- 1 TSP CUMIN SEEDS
- 1/2 TSP TURMERIC
- 1 TSP CUMIN POWDER
- 1/2 TSP CORIANDER POWDER
- 1/2 TSP OF RED CHILI FLAKES
- A PINCH OF BLACK PEPPER TO TASTE
- 2 TBSP COCONUT OIL
- 1 TBSP FRESH CILANTRO, CHOPPED TO GARNISH

In a skillet, add the oil and heat on a medium heat.

Add the black mustard seeds, cumin seeds, and the spices and stir for 4-5 minutes.

Add the onions and stir for a further 5 minutes or until softened.

Add the ginger, garlic and red chili flakes, stirring for a further 5 minutes.

Now add the broccoli rabe and cauliflower to the mix.

Stir until the greens are covered in the spices and then reduce the heat and sauté for about 5-6 minutes.

Garnish with cilantro and add pepper to taste and serve.

BOK CHOY & SESAME SEED STIR FRY

SERVES 2   PREP TIME: 2 MINUTES   COOK TIME: 6 MINUTES

This is another simple stir-fry recipe with bok choy.

- 1 TBSP COCONUT OIL
- 2 CLOVES GARLIC, MINCED
- 1 THUMB SIZED PIECE FRESH GINGER, MINCED
- 4 BOK CHOY PLANTS, LEAVES SEPARATED
- 1 TBSP SESAME SEEDS

Heat the oil in a skillet on a high heat and add in the garlic and ginger. Cook for 1 minute.

Add in thebok choy and cook for about 5 minutes or until the bok choy stalks are crispy.

Season with pepper as needed and sprinkle sesame seeds over to serve.

BEAN SPROUT & TOFU STIR FRY

SERVES 2   PREP TIME: 10 MINUTES   COOK TIME: 20 MINUTES

Easy yet scrumptious mid-week meal.

- 1/2 CUP SOFT TOFU
- 1 GARLIC CLOVE, MINCED
- 1 TBSP FRESH LIME JUICE
- 1 TBSP CANOLA OIL
- 1 CUP FRESH BROCCOLI FLORETS
- 1 TSP BLACK PEPPER
- 1/4 CUP BEANSPROUTS
- 1 CUP COOKED BUCKWHEAT NOODLES

Cut the tofu into cubes and soak the vegetables in warm water.

Heat a skillet on a medium to high heat and add the oil.

Once hot, add the tofu to the skillet and cook for 7-8 minutes or until golden brown.

Add the noodles, bean sprouts and broccoli and sauté for 7-8 minutes or until crisp.

Add the fresh lime juice.

Enjoy!

SPICED SQUASH STEW

SERVES 2   PREP TIME: 10 MINUTES   COOK TIME: 40 MINUTES

A hearty, chunky dish packed full with flavor.

- 1 TBSP EXTRA VIRGIN OLIVE OIL
- 1 ONION, DICED
- 1 GARLIC CLOVE, CHOPPED
- 1/2 STALK CELERY, CHOPPED
- 1 TSP BLACK PEPPER
- 1 TSP TURMERIC
- 1 TSP CUMIN
- 1 TSP GINGER, GRATED
- 1/2 CUP FRESH TOMATOES (OPTIONAL)
- 1/2 CUP HOMEMADE VEG STOCK
- 2 TBSP FRESH CILANTRO
- 1 CUP SPAGHETTI SQUASH
- 1 CUP WATER

In a large pot, heat the oil over a medium to high heat.

After 5 minutes, turn the heat down and sprinkle with spices and ginger.

Now add garlic and celery and continue to sauté for 5 minutes.

Add the tomatoes and stock along with half the cilantro and simmer.

Meanwhile prepare the squash by peeling and chopping into cubes.

Add the squash to the pan and continue to cook for 30 minutes, stirring occasionally.

Scatter with the rest of the cilantro to serve.

VEGETABLE PAELLA

SERVES 2   PREP TIME: 10 MINUTES   COOK TIME: 25 MINUTES

Herby and fresh - amazing!

---

1 CUP LEEK, CHOPPED	1/2 LEMON
1 TBSP EXTRA VIRGIN OLIVE OIL	1 TSP CUMIN
1/2 ZUCCHINI, CHOPPED	1 TSP OREGANO (DRIED)
1/2 RED ONION, CHOPPED	1 TSP PARSLEY (DRIED)
1 CUP BROWN RICE	1 CUP LOW-SALT VEGETABLE BROTH

Add rice to a pot of cold water and cook for 15 minutes.

Drain the water, cover the pan and leave to one side.

Heat the oil in a skillet and add the leek, onion and zucchini, sautéing for 5 minutes.

To the skillet, add the rice, herb, spices and juice of the lemon along with the vegetable stock/water.

Cover and turn heat right down and allow to simmer for 15-20 minutes.

Serve hot.

NORTH AFRICAN SPAGHETTI SQUASH CURRY

SERVES 2   PREP TIME: 10 MINUTES   COOK TIME: 40 MINUTES

A hearty, chunky dish packed full with flavor.

---

1 TBSP EXTRA VIRGIN OLIVE OIL

1 ONION, DICED

1 GARLIC CLOVE, CHOPPED

1/2 STALK CELERY, CHOPPED

1 TSP BLACK PEPPER

1 TSP TURMERIC

1 TSP CUMIN

In a large pot, heat the oil over a medium to high heat.

After 5 minutes, turn the heat down and sprinkle with spices and ginger.

Now add garlic and celery and continue to sauté for 5 minutes.

Add the stock along with half the cilantro and simmer.

Meanwhile prepare the squash by peeling and chopping into cubes.

Add the squash to the pan and continue to cook for 30 minutes, stirring occasionally.

Scatter with the rest of the cilantro to serve.

RADISH, CHIVE & ASPARAGUS PIZZETTE

SERVES 2   PREP TIME: 10 MINUTES   COOK TIME: 50 MINUTES

Very easy to prepare.

- 1/4 CUP OF TOMATOES
- 4 EGG WHITES
- 2 CRUSHED GARLIC CLOVES
- 1/4 CUP FRESH CHOPPED CHIVES
- 1 1/2 TBSP EXTRA VIRGIN OLIVE OIL
- 1/4 CUP LOW FAT HARD CHEESE
- 5 RADISHES, SLICED
- 1/4 CUP ASPARGUS STEMS

Preheat oven to 350°f/180°c/Gas Mark 4.

Whisk the eggs and chives in a bowl and mix in the tomatoes.

Layer radishes, asparagus, garlic and onion slices in a round baking dish and drizzle with olive oil.

Roast in the oven for 15 minutes.

Pour the tomato and egg mixture over the vegetables in the baking dish.

Bake in the oven for 35-40 minutes, or until the center is cooked through (check with a knife).

Sprinkle crumbled brie over the top and place under the broiler to brown.

Enjoy warm or cooled in the fridge with your favorite side salad.

ZUCCHINI SPAGHETTI

SERVES 2   PREP TIME: 10 MINUTES   COOK TIME: 40 MINUTES

Gloriously healthy homemade pasta with a crunchy topping.

- 4 TURNIPS, PEELED AND CUT INTO FINE SHAVINGS
- 4 ZUCCHINIS, PEELED AND SLICED VERTICALLY TO MAKE NOODLES (USE A SPIRALIZER)
- 1 TSP MAPLE SYRUP
- 1 TSP RED CHILI FLAKES
- 1 TBSP EXTRA VIRGIN OLIVE OIL
- 1/2 CUP ARUGULA
- 1/2 LEMON

Preheat the oven to 350°f/170°c/Gas Mark 4.

Soak the vegetables in warm water prior to cooking.

Spread the turnip slices over a baking tray and drizzle over maple syrup before sprinkling with chilli flakes.

Toss to coat.

Add to the oven for 35-40 minutes or until cooked through and slightly crispy.

Meanwhile, heat a pan of water on a high heat and bring to the boil.

Add the zucchini noodles and turn the heat down to simmer for 3-4 minutes.

Remove from the heat and place in a bowl of cold water immediately.

Serve zucchini noodles with turnip shavings and a drizzle of olive oil on top.

Mix the arugula with the lemon juice and serve on the side.

Enjoy!

INDIAN SPICED CHICKPEAS

SERVES 2   PREP TIME: 5 MINUTES   COOK TIME: 25 MINUTES

This is a spicy, tasty vegetarian Indian dish.

1/2 CAULIFLOWER, FLORETS

1/2 CUP CHICKPEAS, DRAINED

1 ONION, DICED

1 THUMB SIZED PIECE OF GINGER, MINCED

4 GARLIC CLOVES, MINCED

1 TSP BLACK MUSTARD SEEDS

1 TSP CUMIN SEEDS

In a skillet, add the oil and heat on a medium heat.

Add the black mustard seeds, cumin seeds, and the spices and stir for 4-5 minutes.

Add the onions and stir for a further 5 minutes or until softened.

Add the ginger, garlic and red chilli flakes, stirring for a further 5 minutes.

Now add the chickpeas to the mix and cook for 10-15 minutes. Add the cauliflower in the last 5 minutes.

Garnish with cilantro and add pepper to taste and serve.

SALADS

ROASTED BEETROOT, GOATS' CHEESE & EGG SALAD

SERVES 2   PREP TIME: 5 MINUTES   COOK TIME: 25 MINUTES

Beetroot is a super food containing nutrients you rarely find in your five portions a day, plus goats' cheese is naturally anti-inflammatory. Worth a go!

- 1/2 CUP COOKED CHOPPED BEETROOT (NOT IN VINEGAR)
- 2 TBSP EXTRA VIRGIN OLIVE OIL
- JUICE FROM 1 ORANGE
- 1 FREE RANGE EGG
- 2 TBSP LOW FAT GREEK YOGURT
- 1 TSP DIJON MUSTARD
- A FEW STALKS OF DILL, FINELY CHOPPED (FRESH OR DRIED)
- 1/2 CUP OF BABY GEM LETTUCE
- HANDFUL OF WALNUTS
- 1/4 CUP CRUMBLED GOATS CHEESE
- A PINCH BLACK PEPPER

Preheat oven to 200°C/400°F/Gas Mark 6.

Place the beetroot onto a lightly oiled baking tray with the juice from the orange and sprinkle with pepper.

Roast for 20-25 minutes, turning once whilst baking. If it starts to dry out, add a little more olive oil.

Meanwhile, boil a pan of water and add the whole egg.

Turn down the heat and simmer for 8 minutes (4 minutes if you like your yolks runny) then run under cold water to cool. Peel and halve.

Mix the remaining oil, yogurt, mustard and chopped dill together - this is the dressing for your lettuce.

Serve the salad with the beetroot and goats' cheese and walnuts crumbled over the top.

BULGARWHEAT, GOATS' CHEESE & TABBOULEH SALAD

SERVES 2   PREP TIME: 35 MINUTES   COOK TIME: NA

A variation of the traditional tabbouleh salad, this version features goats' cheese for a tasty twist.

- 1/2 CUP OF BULGUR WHEAT, UNCOOKED
- 1 CAN OF CHICKPEAS, DRAINED
- 1/4 CUP GOATS' CHEESE, CRUMBLED
- 8 CHERRY TOMATOES, HALVED (OPTIONAL)
- 1 LEMON, JUICED
- 2 TBSP OF FRESH PARSLEY, FINELY CHOPPED
- 1/4 TSP OF BLACK PEPPER
- 1 RED ONION, SLICED THINLY
- 1/4 CUP TABBOULEH, SPIRALYZED
- 2 CUPS OF WATER, BOILING

Mix buckwheat with boiling water in a large bowl.

Cover and set aside for half an hour before draining.

Combine lemon juice, buckwheat, tabbouleh, goats' cheese, tomatoes, red onion, chick peas, pepper and parsley in a large bowl.

Gently toss to mix well.

Serve.

SPINACH, ORANGE AND CRANBERRY SALAD

SERVES 1   PREP TIME: 5 MINUTES   COOK TIME: NA

Fruity and fun!

- 1 CUP FRESH SPINACH WITH THE LEAVES TRIMMED AND COARSELY CHOPPED
- 1 ORANGE, PEELED AND SLICED
- 1 CUP FRESH CRANBERRIES, CHOPPED
- 2 TBSP RED WINE VINEGAR
- 1 TSP OLIVE OIL
- 2 TSP GINGER, PEELED AND GRATED
- A PINCH OF BLACK PEPPER TO TASTE

Grab a salad bowl and mix the vinegar and olive oil until blended and then add in the cranberries and ginger, adding pepper to taste.

Add the spinach and orange slices to the dressing and then toss to coat.

Chill before serving.

KIPPER & CELERY SALAD

SERVES 2　PREP TIME: 2 MINUTES　COOK TIME: NA

Oily fish are recommended up to 6 times per week on an anti-inflammatory diet and taste delicious with celery.

- 1 CAN OF COOKED KIPPERS
- 1 CELERY STALK, CHOPPED
- 1 TBSP FRESH PARSLEY, CHOPPED
- 1/2 CUP LOW FAT GREEK YOGURT
- 1 LEMON, JUICED
- 1 CLOVE GARLIC, MINCED
- 1 ONION, MINCED

Combine all of the ingredients apart from the kippers into a salad bowl.

Drain the kippers and then toss in the dressing mix.

Chill before serving or serve right away if you're in a rush.

Top tip: If you have mackerel or sardines, this works just as well.

ON-THE-GO TACO SALAD

SERVES 2   PREP TIME: 5 MINUTES   COOK TIME: 30 MINUTES

This salad can be enjoyed on the side or as a ready to eat lunch on the go!

- 1 TBSP EXTRA VIRGIN OLIVE OIL
- 2 SKINLESS CHICKEN BREASTS, CHOPPED
- 2 CARROTS, SLICED
- 1/2 LARGE ONION, CHOPPED
- 2 TSP CUMIN SEEDS
- 1/2 AVOCADO, CHOPPED
- 1 JUICED LIME
- 1/2 CUCUMBER, CHOPPED
- 1/2 CUP FRESH SPINACH, WASHED
- 1 MASON OR KILNER JAR

In a skillet, heat up the oil on a medium heat and then cook the chicken for 10-15 minutes until browned and cooked through.

Remove and place to one side to cool.

Add the carrots and onion and continue to cook for 5-10 minutes or until soft.

Add the cumin seeds in a separate pan on a high heat and toast until they're brown before crushing them in a pestle and mortar or blender.

Put them into the pan with the veggies and turn off the heat.

Add the avocado and lime juice into a food processor and blend until creamy.

Layer the jar with half of the avocado and lime mixture, then the cumin roasted veggies, and then the chicken.

Top with the tomatoes, cucumber spinach and serve immediately or save in the fridge for later.

SIZZLING SALMON & GREEN SALAD

SERVES 2   PREP TIME: 2 MINUTES   COOK TIME: 10 MINUTES

A summer time staple.

- 2 SKINLESS SALMON FILLETS
- 2 CUPS OF SEASONAL GREENS
- 1/2 CUP ZUCCHINI, SLICED
- 1 TBSP BALSAMIC VINEGAR

- 1 TBSP EXTRA VIRGIN OLIVE OIL
- 2 SPRIGS THYME, TORN FROM THE STEM
- 1 LEMON, JUICED

Preheat the broiler to a medium high heat.

Broil the salmon in parchment paper with lemon and pepper for 10 minutes.

Meanwhile, slice the zucchini and sauté with the greens for 4-5 minutes with the oil in a pan on a medium heat.

Build the salad by creating a bed of zucchini and topping with flaked salmon.

Drizzle with balsamic vinegar and sprinkle with thyme.

CUMIN & MANGO CHICKEN SALAD

SERVES 2   PREP TIME: 10 MINUTES   COOK TIME: 20 MINUTES

Spicy and refreshing all at the same time!

- 2 FREE RANGE SKINLESS CHICKEN BREASTS
- 1 TSP OREGANO, FINELY CHOPPED
- 1 GARLIC CLOVE, MINCED
- 1 TSP CHILI FLAKES
- 1 TSP CUMIN
- 1 TSP TURMERIC
- 1 TBSP EXTRA VIRGIN OLIVE OIL
- 1 LIME, JUICED
- 1 CUP MANGO, CUBED
- 1/2 ICEBERG/ROMAINE LETTUCE OR SIMILAR, SLICED

In a bowl mix oil, garlic, herbs and spices with the lime juice.

Add the chicken and marinate for as long as time permits.

When ready to serve, preheat the broiler to a medium high heat.

Add the chicken to a lightly greased baking tray and broil for 15-20 minutes or until cooked through.

Combine the lettuce with the mango in a serving bowl.

Once the chicken is cooked, serve immediately on top of the mango and lettuce.

JAPANESE AVOCADO & SHRIMP SALAD

SERVES 2   PREP TIME: 15 MINUTES   COOK TIME: 10 MINUTES

Miso is a soy product with anti-inflammatory properties. Whilst it is high in sodium, it can be enjoyed as a symptom fighter every now and then. It tastes delicious with avocado or on top of your favorite vegetables.

- 1 GARLIC CLOVE, MINCED
- 2 CUPS OF RAW SHRIMP, WITH THE TAILS REMOVED
- 1/2 TBSP EXTRA VIRGIN OLIVE OIL
- 1/2 TSP CHILI POWDER
- 1/4 TSP CAYENNE
- 1 AVOCADO, SLICED
- 1/2 CUCUMBER, CHOPPED
- 2 CUPS SPINACH OR BABY KALE, WASHED AND CHOPPED
- 1 TBSP CILANTRO, FRESHLY CHOPPED
- 1 TBSP PEANUTS, CRUSHED

FOR THE MISO DRESSING:

- 1 THUMB SIZED PIECE OF FRESH GINGER, FINELY CHOPPED
- 2 TBSP EXTRA VIRGIN OLIVE OIL
- 3 TBSP LIME JUICE
- 2 TBSP AGAVE NECTAR/HONEY
- 1 TBSP WHITE MISO (AVAILABLE FROM MOST GROCERY STORES)
- 1/2 TSP MINCED GARLIC

Heat the oil in a skillet over a medium heat, adding in the garlic and shrimp, and then sprinkle with chili powder and cayenne. Sauté for 8-10 minutes or until shrimp is cooked through.

Cut the avocadoes in half and scoop out the flesh.

Dice the cucumber, and chop the baby spinach/ kale.

Arrange in a bowl with the cooked shrimp.

Put all of the ingredients for the dressing into a food processor until smooth.

Pour over the salad and serve immediately, topping with cilantro and peanuts for an extra crunch.

MACKEREL & BEETROOT SUPER SALAD

SERVES 2   PREP TIME: 5 MINUTES   COOK TIME: 20 MINUTES

Packed full of anti-inflammatory super foods, this is such a tasty lunch for yourself or to impress guests at a dinner party.

- 1 CUP SWEET POTATOES, PEELED
- 12 OZ SMOKED MACKEREL FILLETS, SKIN REMOVED
- 2 GREEN ONIONS, FINELY SLICED
- 1 CUP COOKED BEETROOT, SLICED INTO WEDGES
- 2 TBSPS BUNCH DILL, FINELY CHOPPED
- 2 TBSP OLIVE OIL
- JUICE 1 LEMON, ZEST OF HALF
- 1 TSP CARAWAY SEEDS, CRUSHED USING PESTLE AND MORTAR

Place the potatoes in a small saucepan of boiling water and simmer for 15 minutes on a medium high heat or until fork-tender.

Cool and cut into thick slices.

Flake the mackerel into a bowl and add the cooled potatoes, green onions, beetroot and dill.

In a separate bowl, whisk together the olive oil, lemon juice, caraway seeds and black pepper.

Pour over the salad and toss well to coat.

Scatter over the lemon zest.

Pack into plastic containers and chill for later, or enjoy straight away.

EGG & MIXED BEAN SALAD

SERVES 4   PREP TIME: 30 MINUTES   COOK TIME: 0 MINUTES

Classic American side dish.

- 1/2 CUP OF COOKED BLACK BEANS
- 1/2 CUP OF COOKED CANNELLINI BEANS
- 1/2 CUP OF COOKED KIDNEY BEANS
- 2 HARD-BOILED EGGS, SLICED
- 1 CELERY STICK, CHOPPED
- 2 GREEN ONIONS, CHOPPED
- 8 GREEN OLIVES, PITTED AND SLICED
- 1/2 TSP OF BLACK PEPPER
- 3 TSP EXTRA VIRGIN OLIVE OIL
- 1 TSP DRIED OREGANO

Rinse and drain the beans.

Combine celery, olives, olive oil, herbs and beans in a serving bowl and mix.

Refrigerate for at least 30 minutes.

When ready to serve, add the halved boiled eggs.

Sprinkle over chopped green onions and enjoy.

SUPER TOFU & SPINACH SCRAMBLE

SERVES 2   PREP TIME: 5 MINUTES   COOK TIME: 10 MINUTES

Hot and spicy and fresh, this scramble is great for a mid-week meal!

- 1 PACK EXTRA FIRM TOFU, PRESSED AND CRUMBLED
- 1 TBSP OF EXTRA VIRGIN OLIVE OIL
- 2 STEMS OF SPRING ONION, FINELY CHOPPED
- 1 CUP SPINACH LEAVES
- 1/2 CUP CHERRY TOMATOES, QUARTERED (OPTIONAL)
- 1 CLOVE OF GARLIC, FINELY CHOPPED
- 1 TSP OF LEMON JUICE
- 1 TSP BLACK PEPPER

Heat olive oil in a skillet on a medium heat.

Add the spring onion, tomatoes and garlic and sauté for 3-4 minutes.

Lower the heat and add the tofu, lemon juice, and pepper.

Sauté for 3 to 5 minutes.

Turn the heat off and add the spinach – stir until spinach is wilted.

Transfer to a serving dish and enjoy.

MUSTARD & TARRAGON SWEET POTATO SALAD

SERVES 2   PREP TIME: 5 MINUTES   COOK TIME: 30 MINUTES

A BBQ favorite made the healthy way!

- 2 MEDIUM SIZED SWEET POTATOES, PEELED AND CUBED
- 1/2 CUP OF LOW-FAT GREEK YOGURT
- 2 TBSP OF DIJON MUSTARD
- 1 TBSP DRIED TARRAGON
- 1 BEEF TOMATO, FINELY CHOPPED (RETAIN THE SEEDS) - OPTIONAL
- 1/2 YELLOW PEPPER, FINELY CHOPPED - OPTIONAL
- 1/2 RED ONION, FINELY CHOPPED
- PINCH OF BLACK PEPPER TO TASTE

Boil water in a large pot on a high heat.

Cook the potatoes in the pot for 20 minutes or until tender.

Set aside after draining to cool down.

Combine Dijon mustard, plain yogurt, tarragon, peppers, tomatoes and red onion in a serving bowl.

Add the cooled potatoes and mix well.

Enjoy!

MACKEREL & SWEET POTATO SALAD

SERVES 2   PREP TIME: 5 MINUTES   COOK TIME: 20 MINUTES

A delicious potato salad.

---

1 CUP SWEET POTATOES, PEELED

12 OZ SMOKED MACKEREL FILLETS, SKIN REMOVED

2 GREEN ONIONS, FINELY SLICED

1 CUP COOKED BEETROOT, SLICED INTO WEDGES

2 TBSP BUNCH DILL, FINELY CHOPPED

2 TBSP OLIVE OIL

JUICE 1 LEMON, ZEST OF HALF

1 TSP CARAWAY SEEDS, CRUSHED USING PESTLE AND MORTAR

Place the potatoes in a small saucepan of boiling water and simmer for 15 minutes on a medium high heat or until fork-tender.

Cool and cut into thick slices.

Flake the mackerel into a bowl and add the cooled potatoes, green onions, beetroot and dill.

In a separate bowl, whisk together the olive oil, lemon juice, caraway seeds and black pepper.

Pour over the salad and toss well to coat.

Scatter over the lemon zest.

Pack into plastic containers and chill for later, or enjoy straight away.

GREEN ONION & LEMON BUCKWHEAT SALAD

SERVES 2   PREP TIME: 35 MINUTES   COOK TIME: NA

This is very simple to make and tastes great with chicken, fish or roasted vegetables.

- 1/2 CUP DRY BUCKWHEAT
- 1 BUNCH GREEN ONIONS, FINELY CHOPPED
- 3 TBSP FRESH PARSLEY
- 3 TBSP FRESH MINT
- 1/4 EXTRA VIRGIN CUP OLIVE OIL
- 2 LEMONS
- 1 TSP BLACK PEPPER

Soak the vegetables in warm water.

Meanwhile, wash the buckwheat before adding to a pan of cold water on a medium heat.

Bring to the boil and then reduce heat and simmer for 15-20 minutes or until water is mostly absorbed.

Drain any excess liquid from the buckwheat

Drain the vegetables and add to the buckwheat, mixing well.

Add olive oil, lemon juice, herbs and pepper to the mixture.

Let salad set at room temperature for about an hour to absorb the lemon juice and olive oil before serving.

Refrigerate leftovers in an airtight container for 2-3 days.

SIDES

HOMEMADE MOROCCAN HUMMUS

SERVES 4 PREP TIME: 10 MINUTES COOK TIME: NA

Hummus is a great protein-rich snack straight from the Middle East which is now enjoyed across the world.

FOR THE HUMMUS:
- 1 CAN OF CHICKPEAS
- 2 CLOVES OF GARLIC, MINCED
- 1 TBSP TAHINI PASTE
- 4 TBSP EXTRA VIRGIN OLIVE OIL
- 1 TSP GROUND CUMIN
- 1 TSP TURMERIC
- 1 TSP HARISSA
- 1 TSP SALT
- 1 LEMON, JUICED

TO SERVE:
- 1/8 RED ONION, FINELY CHOPPED
- 1/2 BEEF TOMATO, FINELY CHOPPED
- 1 TSP EXTRA VIRGIN OLIVE OIL

Take all of the ingredients for the hummus and add to a food processor until smooth (leave a little chunky for a rustic finish or add a little water to loosen the consistency if required).

Transfer to a serving dish and create a shallow well in the middle with your spoon.

Top with the mixed red onion and tomato and drizzle with the remaining oil to serve.

Sprinkle with a little black pepper to taste and serve as a dip for your favorite veggies or even as a side with your couscous, quinoa or favorite fish or meat dish.

TARRAGON SWEDE AND CARROT MASH

SERVES 4   PREP TIME: 5 MINUTES   COOK TIME: 15 MINUTES

Try this home comfort – it's exciting mash!

- 4 CARROTS, CHOPPED
- 1/2 SWEDE, CHOPPED
- 3 GARLIC CLOVES, CHOPPED
- 1/4 CUP TARRAGON, FINELY CHOPPED
- 1 TBSP EXTRA VIRGIN OLIVE OIL
- A PINCH OF BLACK PEPPER
- 1 TBSP LOW FAT GREEK YOGURT

Put the carrots, swede and garlic in a large pan of water, bring to the boil, and cook for 12 minutes. Drain.

Add the tarragon and olive oil and season with pepper.

Mash with a potato masher.

Stir in a dollop of low fat Greek yogurt if desired.

Serve and enjoy!

SUPER HEALTHY SWEET POTATO FRIES

SERVES 2   PREP TIME: 5 MINUTES   COOK TIME: 30 MINUTES

A healthy version of a favorite snack – enjoy without the guilt!

- 2 LARGE SWEET POTATOES, CUT INTO THIN STRIPS
- 1 TSP OF CUMIN
- 1 TBSP OF EXTRA VIRGIN OLIVE OIL
- 1/2 TSP OF BLACK PEPPER
- 1/2 TSP OF PAPRIKA
- 1 DASH OF CAYENNE PEPPER

Preheat oven to 375°F/190 °C/Gas Mark 5.

Add the sweet potato strips into a large bowl.

Drizzle with some olive oil.

Sprinkle the rest of the ingredients over the top.

Toss together gently to evenly coat the potatoes.

Get a baking sheet and arrange the coated potatoes into a thin layer.

Bake for around 30 minutes or until cooked through.

Serve.

CAYENNE-SPICED BEANS & SWEET POTATO

SERVES 4   PREP TIME: 5 MINUTES   COOK TIME: 30 MINUTES

This is a healthy and tasty rice dish.

- 1 CAN BLACK BEANS
- 1 CAN CANNELLINI BEANS
- 2 SWEET POTATOES, PEELED & CHOPPED
- 2 MEDIUM CARROTS, SLICED
- 2 CLOVES OF GARLIC, MINCED
- 1/2 ONION, DICED
- 1 CAN CHOPPED TOMATOES
- 1 CUP VEGETABLE BROTH
- 1 TBSP CHILI POWDER
- 1/2 TSP GARLIC POWDER
- 2 TBSP EXTRA VIRGIN OLIVE OIL
- 1 TSP CUMIN
- 1/2 TSP CAYENNE
- 1/2 TSP SALT
- 1/2 TSP BLACK PEPPER

Heat olive oil in a pan over a medium heat.

Sautee garlic and onions for 1-2 minutes.

Add carrots and sweet potatoes for about 6 minutes or until the onions are soft.

Lower heat setting to medium-low, then add the rest of the ingredients.

Cover partially and simmer for around 25 minutes, occasionally stirring to prevent sticking.

Serve.

MEXICAN SPICE INFUSED QUINOA

SERVES 1   PREP TIME: 5 MINUTES   COOK TIME: 30 MINUTES

This is a spicy Mexican side dish.

---

1 TSP OLIVE OIL	1 CHOPPED ONION
1 CAN DICED TOMATOES	2 CLOVES GARLIC, MINCED
1 CHILI PEPPER, DICED	1 TBSP PAPRIKA
1 CUP RINSED QUINOA	2 CUPS LOW-SALT CHICKEN BROTH
1 LIME, JUICED	1 CHOPPED JALAPENO

Put the oil in a skillet and cook the quinoa and onion in the oil for 5 minutes or until the onion becomes translucent.

Add the garlic, jalapeno and pepper and then cook for 4-5 minutes until the garlic is fragrant.

Mix the undrained can of tomatoes with the paprika, and the chicken broth into the garllic and pepper.

Turn up heat to allow to boil, then turn heat down and allow to simmer for about 15-20 minutes, until the liquid reduces.

Stir in the cilantro and lime juice and serve.

TASTY TURNIP CHIPS

SERVES 4   PREP TIME: 5 MINUTES   COOK TIME: 50 MINUTES

So easy and satisfying – you can flavor these turnips with whatever spices you like!

- 1 RUTABAGA, PEELED AND FINELY SLICED
- 1 TURNIP, PEELED AND FINELY SLICED
- 1 TBSP EXTRA VIRGIN OLIVE OIL
- 1 ONION, CHOPPED
- 1 CLOVE GARLIC, MINCED
- 1 TSP BLACK PEPPER
- 1 TSP OREGANO
- 1 TSP PAPRIKA

Heat oven to 375°f/190°c/Gas Mark 5.

Grease a baking tray with the olive oil

Add turnip and rutabaga in a thin layer.

Dust over herbs and spices with an extra drizzle of olive oil.

Bake for 40-50 minutes (turning half way through to ensure even crispiness!)

Serve with your choice of low fat Greek yogurt, tomato sauce or mustard.

GINGER PURPLE SPROUTING BROCCOLI

SERVES 2   PREP TIME: 2 MINUTES   COOK TIME: 10 MINUTES

Packing a punch.

---

2 CUPS OF TENDERSTEM BROCCOLI OR PURPLE SPROUTING BROCCOLI

1 THUMB SIZED PIECE OF GINGER, PEELED AND MINCED

1 TBSP EXTRA VIRGIN OLIVE OIL

Boil water in a medium sized pan and steam the broccoli for about 5 minutes or until tender and crisp.

Drain and transfer to ice cold water to preserve the nutrients.

In a skillet, heat the oil for 30 seconds and then stir-fry the ginger for 15 seconds, mixing in the broccoli, and sauteing for 3 minutes until hot throughout.

Serve as a delicious snack or on the side of your favorite meal.

SPINACH & KALE BREADED BALLS

SERVES 4   PREP TIME: 5 MINUTES   COOK TIME: 30 MINUTES

These can be prepared in advance and then heated to serve and are packed with vitamins and iron.

- 2 CUPS FROZEN OR FRESH SPINACH, THAWED AND CHOPPED
- 1 CUP OF FROZEN OR FRESH KALE, THAWED AND DRAINED
- 1/2 CUP ONION, FINELY CHOPPED
- 1 GARLIC CLOVE, FINELY CHOPPED
- 3 TBSP EXTRA VIRGIN OLIVE OIL
- 2 FREE RANGE EGGS, BEATEN
- 1/2 TSP GROUND THYME
- 1/2 TSP RUBBED DRIED OREGANO
- 1/2 TSP DRIED ROSEMARY
- 1 CUP DRY 100% WHOLEGRAIN BREAD CRUMBS
- 1/2 TSP DRIED OREGANO
- 1 TSP GROUND BLACK PEPPER

Preheat oven to 350°f/170°c/Gas Mark 4.

Line a baking sheet with parchment paper.

In a bowl, mix the olive oil and eggs, adding in the spinach, garlic and onions and tossing to coat.

Add the rest of the ingredients, mixing to blend.

Use the palms of your hands to roll into 1 inch balls and arrange them onto the baking sheet.

Bake for 15 minutes, and then flip the balls over.

Continue to bake for another 15 minutes or until they're golden brown.

Serve with low fat Greek yogurt or on their own.

CARROTS AND TART CHERRY KETCHUP

SERVES 2   PREP TIME: 5 MINUTES   COOK TIME: 30 MINUTES

Sweet and savory - give it a go!

---

5 CARROTS, PEELED AND SLICED | **1/2 CUP DRIED TART CHERRIES**

Boil a pan of water on a high heat.

Boil carrots for 10 minutes and then remove and set aside in a separate bowl.

Add the cherries to the water and cook for a further 10 minutes before draining.

Whizz carrots and cherries up in a blender until pureed.

Serve as a dip or drizzled over a summer salad.

MUSTARD CAULIFLOWER SLICES

SERVES 2   PREP TIME: 5 MINUTES   COOK TIME: 0 MINUTES

Raw cauliflower has double the amount of Vitamin B6 and potassium than cooked cauliflower and tastes amazing.

2 CUPS CAULIFLOWER FLORETS, FINELY SLICED

FOR THE DRESSING:

1 TSP EXTRA VIRGIN OLIVE OIL

1 LEMON, JUICED

1 LARGE GARLIC CLOVE, MINCED

1 TSP WHOLEGRAIN MUSTARD

Get a large salad bowl and combine all of the ingredients.

Serve immediately so that the cauliflower remains crunchy!

CASHEW NUTS & BROCCOLI SNACK

SERVES 4   PREP TIME: 5 MINUTES   COOK TIME: 25 MINUTES

This is a simple and flavorsome salad.

1/2 CUP CASHEWS

1/2 CUP WATER

2 TBSP YELLOW CURRY POWDER

PINCH OF PEPPER

4 CUPS BROCCOLI, SLICED

2 TBSP SUNFLOWER SEEDS

Preheat oven to the highest heat.

Layer the cashew nuts onto a dry baking tray and add to the oven for 5-10 minutes or until nuts start to brown. Turn whilst cooking to ensure even browning.

Remove to cool.

Meanwhile boil a pan of water on a medium heat and add the broccoli.

Cook on a simmer for 5-10 minutes or until cooked through.

Drain and place to one side.

Blend the water, curry powder, pepper and sunflower seeds until smooth.

Crush the cashew nuts on a wooden chopping board or similar, using a sharp knife.

When ready to serve, dress the broccoli with the sesame dressing, and top with roasted cashew nuts.

TUNA AND BLACK OLIVE TAPENADE

SERVES 2   PREP TIME: 5 MINUTES   COOK TIME: 0 MINUTES

I love this quick and easy tapanade which can be served on a bed of salad or as a side dish.

1 GARLIC CLOVE	4 ANCHOVIES
1/2 CUP OF SMALL BLACK OLIVES, DRAINED	1 TBSP DIJON MUSTARD
1/2 CUP CAPERS, RINSED AND DRAINED	2 1/2 TBSP OF EXTRA VIRGIN OLIVE OIL
1 CAN OF TUNA IN SPRING WATER, DRAINED	1 CUP WATERCRESS

Add the olives, garlic, capers, anchovies, Dijon mustard, and 2 tbsp olive oil to a food processor for 30 seconds or until a paste is formed.

Transfer to a separate bowl and add 2 tbsp olive oil - do not stir.

Add the tuna to the tapanade and mix well.

Serve on a bed of watercress.

BRILLIANTLY BEETROOT FLAVOURED KETCHUP

SERVES 2   PREP TIME: 5 MINUTES   COOK TIME: 45 MINUTES

Vibrant and enticing.

- 2 WHOLE BEETROOTS
- 1 JUICED LEMON
- 4 TBSP SUNFLOWER SEEDS, SOAKED OVERNIGHT
- 1 TSP MUSTARD POWDER
- A PINCH OF BLACK PEPPER TO TASTE

Preheat oven 350°F/180 °C/Gas Mark 4.

Bake the beetroot for 30-40 minutes or until tender, and then peel and chop into cubes.

Add the rest of the ingredients and the beetroot into a blender and puree until smooth.

Top tip: You can use prepared beetroot as a shortcut as long as there it contains no added sugar or salt (check the package).

ZAINY ZUCCHINI KETCHUP

SERVES 4   PREP TIME: 15 MINUTES   COOK TIME: 0 MINUTES

A yummy alternative to tomato ketchup!

2 ZUCCHINSI, PEELED AND SLICED	1 TBSP EXTRA VIRGIN OLIVE OIL
1/2 CUP FRESH PARSLEY	1 GARLIC CLOVE, MINCED
2 TBSP LEMON JUICE	A PINCH OF BLACK PEPPER
	2 TBSP CHOPPED WALNUTS

Allow zucchini to dry out a little by slicing and placing on kitchen towel to soak up the moisture for 10 minutes or longer if possible.

Process the zucchini with the rest of the ingredients (apart from the nuts) until smooth.

Fold in the nuts to the mixture and then refrigerate for at least 10 minutes before serving with your favorite crudites or sweet potato fries.

LEMONY TARO DIP

SERVES 2 PREP TIME: 5 MINUTES COOK TIME: 30 MINUTES

This is a great dip for a snack or dinner.

GARLIC CLOVE, PEELED	2 TBSP EXTRA VIRGIN OLIVE OIL
3 CUPS OF TARO (RETAIN THE WATER IT WAS COOKED IN)	1/2 CUP FRESH PARSLEY
	1/2 CUP TOASTED PINENUTS
2 TBSP LEMON JUICE	A PINCH OF BLACK PEPPER

In a blender, process the garlic and then add in the taro, lemon juice, olive oil and the water and blend for about 10 seconds.

Transfer to a serving dish and garnish with the parsley, pine nuts and pepper.

FARRO & TOMATO PILAF

SERVES 4   PREP TIME: 5 MINUTES   COOK TIME: 20 MINUTES

An Indian inspired side dish.

- 1 CUP PEARLED FARRO, RINSED
- 2 CUPS WATER
- 1 CUP TOMATOES, CHOPPED
- 1 PACKAGE FRESH MUSHROOMS, SLICED
- 1 TSP CUMIN
- 1 TSP CHILI POWDER
- 1 TSP TURMERIC
- 1 TBSP CILANTRO
- 1/2 YELLOW SQUASH, CUBED

Add the faro and water to a saucepan and boil on a high heat until boiling.

Reduce the heat, cover and simmer for 20 minutes or until the farro is tender and the liquid is absorbed.

Meanwhile, in a separate pan on a medium heat, cook the tomatoes and mushrooms with the cilantro and spices until the mushrooms are soft (5 minutes).

Add the squash and sauté for 10 minutes or until all of the vegetables are tender.

Drain and stir the farro into the squash mix until heated through.

Serve alone as lunch or on the side of your favorite dish.

RUSTIC APRICOT & WALNUT RICE

SERVES 2   PREP TIME: 5 MINUTES   COOK TIME: 25 MINUTES

A sweet and savory side.

- 1/2 CUP WALNUTS
- 2 CUPS HOMEMADE CHICKEN BROTH
- 1 CUP UNCOOKED BROWN RICE
- 1 TBSP EXTRA VIRGIN OLIVE OIL
- 1 ONION, CHOPPED
- 1/1 CUP DRIED APRICOTS
- 1 ORANGE, ZEST AND JUICE

Preheat oven to 375°F/190 °C/Gas Mark 5.

Layer walnuts on a baking tray and roast for 10 minutes.

Meanwhile, put the broth and brown rice into a saucepan and boil on a high heat.

Reduce the heat and simmer for 25 minutes until rice is cooked and the broth is absorbed.

Meanwhile, heat the oil in a skillet on a medium heat and sauté the onion until soft.

Add the apricots and cook for another 10 minutes.

Stir in the walnuts and the orange zest and juice, and then fold the mixture into the rice, adding pepper to taste.

ROASTED PAPRIKA PUMPKIN SEEDS

SERVES 4   PREP TIME: 5 MINUTES   COOK TIME: 15 MINUTES

Energy boosting bites – great as a topping for cereals or soups, or as a quick pick me up throughout the day!

- 1 CUP PUMPKIN SEEDS
- 1 TBSP EXTRA VIRGIN OLIVE OIL
- 1 TSP PAPRIKA
- 1 TSP CHILI POWDER
- 1 TSP DRIED OREGANO

Preheat oven to 375°F/190 °C/Gas Mark 5.

Layer the seeds on a baking tray.

Combine the oil, paprika, oregano and the chili powder together and coat the pumpkin seeds evenly.

Bake for 15 minutes and serve.

FAST & FRESH GRANOLA TRAIL MIX

SERVES 2   PREP TIME: 5 MINUTES   COOK TIME: 20 MINUTES

This is a tasty granola filled with protein and so much healthier than the shop bought version.

1 CUP TOASTED ALMONDS	1/2 CUP CHERRIES
1 TBSP RAW HONEY	1 CUP GRANOLA

Preheat oven to 350°F/170 °C/Gas Mark 4.

Spread the almonds across a baking sheet.

Bake for five minutes and then add cherries and granola and toss.

Drizzle honey on top and toss again to coat before baking in oven for 10-15 minutes.

Remove to cool.

Serve alone or with your choice of milk as a cereal

BAKED APPLE & WALNUT CHIPS

SERVES 4   PREP TIME: 5 MINUTES   COOK TIME: 30 MINUTES

Another moreish snack that will satisfy your sweet cravings without flaring up your symptoms!

---

4 APPLES, PEELED AND THINLY SLICED

1 TBSP CINNAMON

1/4 CUP OF WALNUT PIECES FOR TOPPING

Preheat oven to 190°C/375°F/Gas Mark 5.

Layer the apple slices in a thin layer on a baking tray.

Dust with the cinnamon and top with walnut pieces.

Bake for 20-30 minutes or until crispy.

SPICED APPLE & QUINCE SAUCE

SERVES 2   PREP TIME: 5 MINUTES   COOK TIME: 40 MINUTES

This is a great fruity side sauce for whole-wheat crackers or celery.

- 2 QUINCES, PEELED, CORED AND DICED
- 4 CUPS COOKING APPLES, CUT INTO CHUNKS
- 1 ORANGE, JUICED
- 1 CINNAMON STICK

Put the quinces and apples in a large pan of water on a medium heat and simmer for 30-40 minutes or until tender (your fork should go right through and crumble the apple).

Add to the blender with the rest of the ingredients and whizz up until pureed.

You can serve hot or cold with your favorite snacks.

LIME & CARROT COLESLAW

SERVES 2   PREP TIME: 15 MINUTES   COOK TIME: 0 MINUTES

Lovely healthy side dish or snack.

- 1 CARROT, PEELED AND FINELY SLICED
- 1 CUP WHITE CABBAGE, PEELED AND FINELY SLICED
- 1 LIME, JUICE AND ZEST
- 1 TBSP FRESH PARSLEY, FINELY CHOPPED
- 1 TBSP EXTRA VIRGIN OLIVE OIL

Soak vegetables in warm water for 5-10 minutes.

Drain and rinse with cold water.

Combine with the rest of the ingredients, cover and cool in refrigerator before serving.

RAINBOW RICE SALAD

SERVES 2   PREP TIME: 10 MINUTES   COOK TIME: 35 MINUTES

Tasty and aesthetic rice side dish.

- 1 TBSP EXTRA VIRGIN OLIVE OIL
- 1 TBSP BALSAMIC VINEGAR
- 1 TSP BLACK PEPPER
- 1 GARLIC CLOVE, MINCED
- 1 TSP DRIED BASIL
- 1 TSP DRIED OREGANO
- 1 TSP FRESH PARSLEY
- 1/2 RED ONION, DICED
- 1/4 CUCUMBER, PEELED AND DICED
- 1 1/2 CUPS COOKED WILD RICE
- 1/2 CUP FROZEN GREEN BEANS, CHOPPED

Add all of the ingredients to a bowl and toss to coat (ensure cooked rice is completely cool).

Add to an airtight container and store in the fridge for up to 2 days.

Serve cold.

CHILI & LEMON QUINOA

SERVES 2   PREP TIME: 5 MINUTES   COOK TIME: 30 MINUTES

A great addition to any meal.

---

1 TSP OLIVE OIL

1 CUP RINSED QUINOA

1 LEMON, JUICED

1 CHOPPED ONION

2 CUPS HOMEMADE CHICKEN BROTH

1 CHOPPED JALAPENO

2 TBSP CILANTRO

Put the oil in a skillet and cook the quinoa and onion in the oil for 5 minutes or until the onion becomes translucent.

Add the jalapeño and cook for 4-5 minutes.

Add the chicken broth to the pan.

Turn up heat to allow to boil, then turn heat down and allow to simmer for about 15-20 minutes, until the liquid reduces.

Stir in the cilantro and lemon juice and serve.

CAULIFLOWER COUSCOUS

SERVES 2   PREP TIME: 5 MINUTES   COOK TIME: 20 MINUTES

Spicy and delicious side dish.

---

2 TBSP EXTRA VIRGIN OLIVE OIL

1/4 CAULIFLOWER

1 LEMON, JUICE & ZEST

1 TSP CURRY POWDER

1/4 RED ONION, FINELY DICED

Soak vegetables in warm water prior to use.

Grate the cauliflower with a cheese grater.

In a large bowl, add cauliflower, red onion, lemon juice and curry powder.

Use your hands to toss the mixture and top with a little lemon zest to serve.

Refrigerate before serving or eat up straight away!

SPICED PUMPKIN PANCAKES

SERVES 2   PREP TIME: 5 MINUTES   COOK TIME: 6 MINUTES

A great go-to made with your pantry essentials.

- 1 CUP OF CANNED PUMPKIN, NO ADDED SALT OR SUGAR
- 2 TBSP WATER
- 3 EGG WHITES
- 1 TBSP COCONUT OIL
- 1 TSP CAYENNE PEPPER
- 1 TSP CINNAMON

Blend the pumpkin flesh together with water to form a smooth pulp.

Now add the rest of the ingredients (minus the coconut oil) and mix well.

Heat a large pan with coconut oil.

Pour the pumpkin mixture into the pan into individual rounded pancakes (go easy at first and pour your mixture into little circles, keep pouring whilst tilting the pan until you have a pancake to your desired shape).

Lift the mixture with a spatula and then flip. Cook for 3 minutes on either side.

Serve warm - they taste great with sweet or savory accompaniments.

MEXICAN SALSA

SERVES 2   PREP TIME: 10 MINUTES   COOK TIME: 35 MINUTES

Refreshing and vibrant.

1/4 RED ONION, FINELY DICED	1/4 CUP MANGO/PINEAPPLE, DICED
1 LIME, JUICED	1 TBSP FRESH CILANTRO, FINELY CHOPPED
1/2 LEMON, JUICED	
1 TSP WHITE VINEGAR	
1 TSP BLACK PEPPER	

Soak vegetables in warm water.

Combine all ingredients in a bowl and toss to coat.

Store in an airtight container in the fridge for 2-3 days or serve right away.

Use on the side of fish, meats, tacos or salads.

WATERCRESS, LEMON & CRANBERRY SALAD

SERVES 2   PREP TIME: 5 MINUTES   COOK TIME: 0 MINUTES

Fruity fun and fast!

- 1 CUP FRESH WATERCRESS
- 1 LEMON, PEELED AND SLICED
- 1/2 CUP FRESH CRANBERRIES
- 2 TBSP BALSAMIC VINEGAR
- 4 TSP EXTRA VIRGIN OLIVE OIL
- 2 TSP FRESH GINGER, PEELED AND GRATED
- A PINCH OF BLACK PEPPER TO TASTE

Grab a salad bowl and mix the vinegar and olive oil until blended and then add in the cranberries, ginger and pepper to taste

Add the watercress and lemon juice to the dressing, and then toss to coat.

Chill for 15 minutes before serving.

DESSERTS

WALNUT & DARK CHOCOLATE CHIP COOKIES

SERVES 5   PREP TIME: 10 MINUTES   COOK TIME: 10 MINUTES

These wholegrain cookies are just as delicious as their sugary companions! .

- 1 CUP WALNUTS/PECANS
- 1 CUP GROUND FLAX MEAL
- 2 CUPS WHOLEGRAIN ROLLED OATS
- 1 TSP CINNAMON
- 1/2 CUP WHOLEWHEAT FLOUR
- 1 TSP BAKING SODA

- 1/4 CUP STEVIA
- 1 FREE RANGE EGG
- 1/4 CUP CANOLA OIL
- 1 TSP VANILLA EXTRACT
- 1 CUP DARK CHOCOLATE CHIPS
- 1/2 CUP DRIED TART CHERRIES
- 1/2 CUP WHOLE ALMOND BUTTER

Preheat the oven to 190°C/375°F/Gas Mark 5.

Line a baking dish with parchment paper.

Grind the walnuts in a blender to make flour.

Add all of the other ingredients (except for the almond butter, cherries and chocolate chips) and process.

Add mixture to a bowl and then fold in the chocolate chips and cherries.

Mix the flour mixture into the almond butter until a sticky dough is formed.

Use a tablespoon to spoon mini cookie shapes onto your baking tray and bake for 9 minutes before placing them on a wire rack to cool.

STRAWBERRY AND BANANA PUDDING

SERVES 2   PREP TIME: 30 MINUTES   COOK TIME: 5 MINS

Summery and scrumptious!

---

1 CUP OF STRAWBERRIES, SLICED

1/4 CUP OF FREE RANGE EGG WHITES

4 SQUARES DARK COOKING CHOCOLATE

1 SMALL BANANA, SLICED

1/2 CUP BLUEBERRIES

2 TBSP OF WATER

Melt the dark chocolate over a bowl of boiling water on a low heat on the stove.

Add the water and egg whites to the melted chocolate and mix well to reach a thick consistency.

Spoon the batter out onto a small plate.

Put in the freezer for half an hour.

Garnish with the strawberries, banana and blueberries to serve.

VANILLA AND NUTMEG MUFFINS WITH BLUEBERRIES

SERVES 4　PREP TIME: 5 MINUTES　COOK TIME: 20 MINUTES

Scrumptious muffins to be enjoyed as a delicious dessert or breakfast!

- 3 FREE RANGE EGG WHITES
- 1/10 CUP CHICKPEA FLOUR
- 1 TBSP COCONUT FLOUR
- 1 TSP OF BAKING POWDER
- 1 TBSP NUTMEG, GRATED
- 1 TSP VANILLA EXTRACT
- 1 TSP STEVIA
- 1/2 CUP FRESH BLUEBERRIES

Pre-heat the oven to 325°F/170 °C/Gas Mark 3.

Mix all of the ingredients in a mixing bowl.

Divide the batter into 4 and spoon into a muffin tin.

Bake in the oven for 15-20 minutes or until cooked through.

Your knife should pull out clean from the middle of the muffins once done.

Allow to cool on a wired rack before serving.

HOMEMADE HOT CROSS BUNS

SERVES 8   PREP TIME: 5 MINUTES   COOK TIME: 20 MINUTES

Anti-inflammatory friendly treats.

- 3 CUPS ALMONDS
- 1 CUP RAISINS
- 1 TBSP RAW HONEY
- ZEST AND JUICE OF 1 ORANGE AND 1 LEMON
- 1 TSP CINNAMON
- 1 TSP CLOVES
- 1 TSP NUTMEG

Lightly oil a muffin tray.

Whizz up the almonds into a powder in a food processor.

Add the honey, spices, lemon juice and orange juice and process until you have a dough.

You can then blend in the raisins and the fruit zest for about 30 seconds.

Divide mixture into eight in the muffin tray and then cross the top of each bun with a sharp knife.

Add to the oven for 15-20 minutes or until risen and cooked through.

These should be served immediately and enjoyed with your favorite fresh fruit.

CINEMA SWEET AND SALTY NUTS

SERVES 4　　PREP TIME: 2 MINUTES　　COOK TIME: 20 MINUTES

Fill your stomachs with a guilt-free indulgent treat.

---

2 CUPS OF UNSALTED MIXED NUTS – PECANS, PEANUTS AND ALMONDS

1 FREE RANGE EGG WHITE

1 TBSP HONEY

1 TSP COCONUT OIL FOR COOKING

1 TSP BLACK PEPPER

1 PINCH CHILI POWDER

Preheat oven to 375°F/190 °C/Gas Mark 5.

In a pan add the egg white, chili, pepper and honey and heat on a low heat for 3 minutes.

Put the nuts into the pan and then coat them with the mixture.

Once ready, spread the nuts into a single layer on a baking sheet and then bake for at least 15 minutes.

Be careful they don't burn by turning half way through.

Remove and cool before serving.

SPICED ORANGES

SERVES 2   PREP TIME: 20 MINUTES   COOK TIME: 15 MINUTES

These oranges are great in the winter or on a hot summer's day!

1/2 CUP WATER	1 SMALL CINNAMON STICK
1 TBSP RAW HONEY	1 CLOVE
1 LEMON	2 ORANGES, PEELED AND SECTIONED
	1 SPRIG OF FRESH MINT

Add all of the ingredients (minus the oranges) to a saucepan.

Cook over a medium heat until thickened (10-15 minutes).

Add the oranges, and then simmer for 1 minute.

Transfer all ingredients to a bowl or container and place in the fridge, marinating for at least 2 hours or preferably overnight.

Drain orange slices and garnish with a little more fresh mint to serve.

Best served with low fat Greek yogurt for summer or warmed through in the winter.

FRUIT COCKTAIL WITH ROSE WATER YOGURT

SERVES 4   PREP TIME: 10 MINUTES   COOK TIME: 0 MINUTES

A timeless treat!

- 1 TBSP ROSE WATER (AVAILABLE IN MOST EXOTIC AISLES IN GROCERY STORES, ALTERNATIVELY USE 1-2 DROPS OF ROSE OIL)
- 2 CUPS FRESH STRAWBERRIES, HALVED
- 2 PLUMS, PITTED AND CUBED
- 2 KIWIS, PEELED AND CUBED
- 1 PEACH, PEELED AND CUBED
- 1 CUP HONEYDEW MELON, PEELED AND CUBED
- 1 CUP OF TART CHERRIES, PITTED AND HALVED
- 1 CUP GRAPES, HALVED
- 1 CUP FRESH PINEAPPLE, CUBED
- 2 CUPS LOW-FAT GREEK YOGURT (OPTIONAL)

Add all of the fruit to a mixing bowl and stir.

In a separate bowl, add rose water to yogurt and stir.

Divide fruit into 4 servings and top with rose water yogurt.

Enjoy!

DATE COMPOTE

SERVES 2   PREP TIME: 5 MINUTES   COOK TIME: 30 MINUTES

Rich and satisfying.

---

2 CUPS OF DATES, FINELY CHOPPED	2 CUPS DRIED PEACHES, FINELY CHOPPED
2 CUPS DRIED APRICOTS, FINELY CHOPPED	4 CUPS APPLES,
2 CUPS BLACK FIGS, FINELY CHOPPED	1 LEMON

Add fruit to a large pot and cover with water.

Soak the fruit for an hour and then bring to a boil on a high heat.

Turn down the heat and simmer for 5 minutes.

Add the juice of 1 lemon and stir.

Remove from the heat and allow to cool.

Whizz up in the blender if needed to smooth any lumps.

Serve warm on the side of any dessert or as a dip or accompaniment to bread/crackers/vegetables.

FRUIT PUDDING

SERVES 2   PREP TIME: 5 MINUTES   COOK TIME: 30 MINUTES

Tropical and delicious.

- 15 APRICOTS
- 10 PRUNES
- 6 FREE RANGE EGGS
- 3 CUPS WATER
- 1 CUP RAW PECANS/WALNUTS
- 2 TBSP PURE VANILLA EXTRACT
- 2 BROKEN CINNAMON STICKS

Preheat oven to 180°C/350°F/Gas Mark 4.

In a large saucepan, boil the water on a high heat and then add the apricots, prunes, cinnamon sticks before turning down the heat and simmering for 30 minutes.

Allow to cool.

Remove the cinnamon sticks and blend in a blender or food processor, adding in the eggs and vanilla until smooth.

Add mixture to a glass oven dish and layer the top with the nuts.

Oven bake for 30 minutes.

Cool and serve.

Top tip: this recipe contains 6 eggs so ensure this is best shared so as not to go over your protein recommendations!

GRILLED BANANA AND NUT BUTTER

SERVES 2   PREP TIME: 5 MINUTES   COOK TIME: 30 MINUTES

Loaded with goodness for a mid afternoon snack!

3 BANANAS	3 TBSP ORGANIC ALMOND BUTTER (CHECK LABEL TO ENSURE THERE ARE NO EXTRA INGREDIENTS)

Split a banana lengthways with a knife down to its centre to form a banana split.

Spread almond butter along the middle and broil for 3-4 minutes under broiler on a medium heat until browned.

Serve immediately – this is just as tasty cold if you're in a rush!

APRICOT AND COCONUT WHOLEFOOD BITES

SERVES 2   PREP TIME: 5 MINUTES   COOK TIME: 30 MINUTES

Healthy and sweet breakfast or snack bites.

SUN-DRIED APRICOTS, FINELY CHOPPED

RAW WALNUTS OR PECANS, FINELY CHOPPED

1/2 CUP DESICCATED COCONUT

1 TBSP HONEY

Mix the ingredients together to form a sticky dough.

Shape it into bite size balls with the palms of your hands.

Cover and refrigerate for at least 2 hours to set.

Serve or wrap for later.

COCONUT, BANANA AND RASPBERRY HOT MILK

SERVES 2   PREP TIME: 5 MINUTES   COOK TIME: 30 MINUTES

A hot drink full of fruity flavor.

---

1 CAN LOW FAT COCONUT MILK

3 BANANAS, SLICED

1/2 CUP FRESH RASPBERRIES

In a pan simmer ingredients for 10 minutes on a medium-low heat.

Whizz up in a blender until smooth.

Serve warm or allow to cool and add ice cubes to serve as a chilled milkshake.

SPICED PUMPKIN PANCAKES

SERVES 2   PREP TIME: 5 MINUTES   COOK TIME: 30 MINUTES

Slightly savory pancakes for the lesser of the sweet tooths amongst us!

FLESH FROM 1/4 DESEEDED PUMPKIN

4 EGGS (FREE RANGE)

3 EGG WHITES (FREE RANGE)

SPRINKLE OF BLACK PEPPER

1/2 TSP GLUTEN-FREE BAKING SODA

2 TBSP COCONUT OIL

1 TBSP GOOD QUALITY MAPLE SYRUP (NOT THE COMMERCIAL STUFF FOUND IN BIG SUPERMARKETS – TRY LOCAL SHOPS/FARM SHOPS TO ENSURE YOU'RE STICKING TO PALEO!)

1 HANDFUL PECAN NUTS

In a blender or food processor, blend the pumpkin flesh together with some water to form a smooth pulp.

Now add the eggs, freshly ground pepper, 1 tbsp of coconut oil, and a tiny pinch of baking soda to the pumpkin mix and blend until smooth.

Heat a large pan on a medium heat with the other 1 tbsp of coconut oil.

Pour into the pan individual rounded pancakes (go easy at first and pour your mixture into little circles, keep pouring whilst tilting the pan until you have a pancake to your desired shape).

Lift the mixture with a spatula and then flip.

Cook for 3 minutes on either side.

Plate and serve with pecan nuts and maple syrup.

PEANUT CEREAL BARS

SERVES 2　PREP TIME: 5 MINUTES　COOK TIME: 30 MINUTES

Save your money with these homemade cereal bars - they're delicious!

---

2 CUPS OF WHOLEGRAIN OATS

1 CUP ALMOND BUTTER (WHOLEFOOD – NO ADDED SUGAR OR SALT OR OILS)

1/2 CUP COCONUT MILK

Get a bowl and add the coconut milk and whisk until smooth.

Add the peanut butter and mix thoroughly.

Pour the oats into the bowl and again mix through.

Scoop out the mixture into a baking tray and flatten until the surface is smooth.

Place the tray in the fridge and leave for around 8 hours.

Cut into bars.

FRUIT AND NUT SLICES

SERVES 2   PREP TIME: 5 MINUTES   COOK TIME: 30 MINUTES

Sweet and savory treat.

---

1 TBSP DRIED DATES, DICED

1 TBSP DRIED CRANBERRIES

1 TBSP COCONUT FLAKES

1 TBSP WALNUTS/PECANS, GROUND

Mix all of the ingredients in a bowl.

Use your hands to shape the mixture into a ball.

Lay out tin foil and then flatten and roll the mixture with the palms of your hands to form a cylinder shape.

Roll and wrap in the tinfoil and then leave it in the fridge for 30 minutes until it hardens before slicing into disk shape slices and serving with some fresh fruit or yogurt.

PEANUT CHOCOLATE PANCAKES

SERVES 2 PREP TIME: 5 MINUTES COOK TIME: 10 MINUTES

Much better than your average candy bar.

- 2 TBSP OF SMOOTH PEANUT BUTTER (WHOLEFOOD – NO ADDED SUGAR OR SALT OR OILS)
- 2 SQUARES OF DARK CHOCOLATE, GRATED
- 2 FREE RANGE EGG WHITES
- 2 TBSP OF RAW COCONUT FLOUR
- 1 TBSP COCONUT OIL

Get a bowl and combine all the ingredients.

Mix well to form a thick batter.

Heat a skillet on a medium heat and add the coconut oil.

Pour half the mixture onto the center of the pan, to form a pancake and cook through for 3-4 minutes on each side.

Serve with your choice of berry or Greek yogurt and the gratings of dark chocolate for an indulgent treat.

LEMON LAVENDER & STRAWBERRY COMPOTE

SERVES 4   PREP TIME: 5 MINUTES   COOK TIME: 30 MINUTES

So sweet and delicious.

2 CUPS OF STRAWBERRIES, HALVED	2 TBSP RAW HONEY
JUICE AND ZEST OF 1 LEMON	1 TBSP LAVENDER EXTRACT

Put all of the ingredients together into a saucepan and then simmer on a very low heat until the honey has been dissolved (15-20 minutes).

When the sauce starts to thicken, add the strawberries and simmer for 5-10 minutes.

Serve warm right away or allow to cool and drizzle over yogurt later on.

PECAN & DATE SNACK BARS

SERVES 4   PREP TIME: 20 MINUTES   COOK TIME: 40 MINUTES

These are great protein bars for on the go healthy snacking!

---

4 CUPS OF DATES, PITTED AND CHOPPED

3 CUPS PECANS

Preheat the oven to 180°C/350°F/Gas Mark 4.

Put the dates in a bowl and cover them with water.

Leave for at least 20 minutes and then blitz the pecans in a food processor until they form a 'breadcrumb' texture.

Now, drain the water from the dates and then add to the processor until the nuts and fruit create a dough that easily needs together with your hands.

Line a baking sheet with parchment paper and then spread the dough onto the pan into a layer 2 inches thick.

Bake for 35-40 minutes or until cooked through and crispy on the top.

Remove to cool and slice into bars to serve.

SUNSHINE CEREAL BITES

SERVES 2   PREP TIME: 20 MINUTES   COOK TIME: 30 MINUTES

You can't stay dreary and sad with these delectable fruit bites!

---

1 CUP UNSWEETENED PINEAPPLE, DRIED

1/2 CUP WARM WATER

1 CUP CASHEWS

1/2 CUP COCONUT FLAKES

1/2 TSP LEMON ZEST

1 TBSP HONEY

Preheat oven to 190°C/375°F/Gas Mark 5.

Soak the pineapple slices in warm water for 20 minutes until softened.

Combine with the rest of the ingredients and mix.

Spread onto a lined baking tray and bake for 20-30 minutes or until crispy.

PECAN & MAPLE SYRUP COOKIES

SERVES 2   PREP TIME: 10 MINUTES   COOK TIME: 10 MINUTES

Superb!

- 1/4 CUP PECANS
- 1/4 CUP GROUND FLAX MEAL
- 1/2 CUP GLUTEN-FREE ROLLED OATS
- 1 TSP CINNAMON
- 1/4 CUP WHOLEWHEAT FLOUR
- 1 TSP BAKING SODA
- 1 TBSP STEVIA
- 1 FREE RANGE EGG
- 2 TBSP CANOLA OIL
- 1 TSP VANILLA EXTRACT
- 1/4 CUP MAPLE SYRUP
- 4 TBSP DRIED TART CHERRIES
- 4 TBSP WHOLE ALMOND BUTTER

Preheat the oven to 190°C/375°F/Gas Mark 5.

Line a baking dish with parchment paper.

Grind the pecans in a blender to make flour.

Add all of the other ingredients (except for the almond butter, cherries) and process.

Add mixture to a bowl and then fold in the cherries.

Mix the flour mixture into the almond butter until a sticky dough is formed.

Use a tablespoon to spoon mini cookie shapes onto your baking tray and bake for 9 minutes before placing them on a wire rack to cool.

LEMON & SUNFLOWER SEED MUFFINS WITH RASPBERRIES

SERVES 2   PREP TIME: 5 MINUTES   COOK TIME: 20 MINUTES

Scrumptious muffins to be enjoyed as a delicious dessert or breakfast!

- 2 FREE RANGE EGG WHITES
- 2 TBSP CHICKPEA FLOUR
- 1/2 TBSP COCONUT FLOUR
- 1 TSP OF BAKING POWDER
- 1 TBSP NUTMEG, GRATED
- 1 TSP VANILLA EXTRACT
- 1 TSP STEVIA
- 1/2 LEMON, ZESTED
- 1 TBSP SUNFLOWER SEEDS
- 1/2 CUP FRESH RASPBERRIES

Pre-heat the oven to 325°F/170 °C/Gas Mark 3.

Mix all of the ingredients in a mixing bowl.

Divide the batter into 4 and spoon into a muffin tin.

Bake in the oven for 15-20 minutes or until cooked through.

Your knife should pull out clean from the middle of the muffins once done.

Allow to cool on a wired rack before serving.

TOASTED FRUIT CAKES

SERVES 2   PREP TIME: 5 MINUTES   COOK TIME: 20 MINUTES

Anti-inflammatory friendly treats.

- 1/2 CUP ALMONDS
- 1 TBSP RAW HONEY
- ZEST AND JUICE OF 1 LEMON
- 1 TSP CINNAMON
- 1 TSP CLOVES
- 1 TSP NUTMEG
- 1 BANANA, SLICED

Lightly oil a muffin tray.

Whiz up the almonds into a powder in a food processor.

Add the honey, spices, lemon juice and process until you have a dough.

You can then blend in the banana and the fruit zest for about 30 seconds.

Divide mixture into eight in the muffin tray and then cross the top of each bun with a sharp knife.

Add to the oven for 15-20 minutes or until risen and cooked through.

These should be served immediately and enjoyed with your favorite fresh fruit.

SPICED PEACHES

SERVES 2   PREP TIME: 5 MINUTES   COOK TIME: 10 MINUTES

These are so easy to prepare and impress every time.

---

1 CUP CANNED PEACHES IN THEIR OWN JUICES

1 TSP GROUND CLOVES

1 TSP GROUND CINNAMON

1 TSP GROUND NUTMEG

ZEST OF 1/2 LEMON

1/2 CUP WATER

Drain peaches.

Combine water, cinnamon, nutmeg, ground cloves and lemon zest in a pan on the stove.

Heat on a medium heat and add peaches.

Bring to a boil, reduce the heat and simmer for 10 minutes.

Serve warm.

COCONUT PANCAKES

SERVES 2   PREP TIME: 5 MINUTES   COOK TIME: 10 MINUTES

Tropical dessert.

- 2 FREE RANGE EGG WHITES
- 2 TBSP COCONUT FLOUR
- 3 TBSP COCONUT SHAVINGS
- 2 TBSP COCONUT MILK (OPTIONAL)
- 1 TBSP COCONUT OIL

Get a bowl and combine all the ingredients.

Mix well until you get a thick batter.

Heat a skillet on a medium heat and heat the coconut oil.

Pour half the mixture to the center of the pan, forming a pancake and cook through for 3-4 minutes on each side.

Serve with your choice of berries on the top.

COCONUT & CRANBERRY BARS

SERVES 2   PREP TIME: 5 MINUTES   COOK TIME: 30 MINUTES

Sweet and savory treat.

- 1 TBSP DRIED DATES, DICED
- 1 TBSP DRIED CRANBERRIES
- 1 TBSP COCONUT FLAKES
- 1 TBSP WALNUTS/PECANS, GROUND

Mix all of the ingredients in a bowl.

Use your hands to shape the mixture into a ball.

Lay out tin foil and then flatten and roll the mixture with the palms of your hands to form a cylinder shape.

Roll and wrap in the tinfoil and then leave it in the fridge for 30 minutes until it hardens before slicing into disk shape slices and serving with some fresh fruit or yogurt.

APPENDIX
CONVERSION TABLES

Volume

Imperial	Metric
1 tbsp	15ml
2 fl oz	55 ml
3 fl oz	75 ml
5 fl oz (¼ pint)	150 ml
10 fl oz (½ pint)	275 ml
1 pint	570 ml
1 ¼ pints	725 ml
1 ¾ pints	1 litre
2 pints	1.2 litres
2½ pints	1.5 litres
4 pints	2.25 litres

Oven temperatures

Gas Mark	Fahrenheit	Celsius
1/4	225	110
1/2	250	130
1	275	140
2	300	150
3	325	170
4	350	180
5	375	190
6	400	200
7	425	220
8	450	230
9	475	240

Weight

Imperial	Metric
½ oz	10 g
¾ oz	20 g
1 oz	25 g
1½ oz	40 g
2 oz	50 g
2½ oz	60 g
3 oz	75 g
4 oz	110 g
4½ oz	125 g
5 oz	150 g
6 oz	175 g
7 oz	200 g
8 oz	225 g
9 oz	250 g
10 oz	275 g

BIBLIOGRAPHY

Beck, S. (2013) Acute and Chronic Information. [online] Hopkins Medicine. Available at: http://www.hopkinsmedicine.org/mcp/education/300.713%20lectures/300.713%202013/beck_08.26.2013.pdf Accessed 03/04/2016

Women's Health, (2012). Auto-immune Diseases Fact Sheet. Available at: http://www.womenshealth.gov/publications/our-publications/fact-sheet/autoimmune-diseases.html#a Accessed 04/03/2016

MACKAY, I AND ROSEN, F. (2001) Autoimmune Diseases. The New England Journal of Medicine [online] Vol. 345, No. 5, · www.nejm.org. [Accessed 07/02/2016]

US National Library of Medicine (2014) Multiple Sclerosis. Available at: https://www.nlm.nih.gov/medlineplus/ency/article/000737.htm [Accessed 04/03/2016]

Cosentino, F and Assenza, E. (December 2004), Diabetes and Inflammation. Herz. Volume 29, Issue 8, pp 749-759 [Accessed 07/02/2016]

Baecklund, E and Anastasia, L. (February 2006), Arthritis & Rheumatism. Volume 54, Issue 3, pages 692–701, [Accessed 07/02/2016]
Xu, Haiyan et al. "Chronic Inflammation In Fat Plays A Crucial Role In The Development Of Obesity-Related Insulin Resistance". Journal of Clinical Investigation 112.12 (2003): 1821-1830. Web. [Accessed 07/02/2016]

Shacter, E and Weitzman, SA (2002) Chronic inflammation and cancer. Oncology (Williston Park, N.Y.) Volume 16, Issue 2. pp. 217-26, 229 [Accessed 07/02/2016]

Galland, L. "Diet And Inflammation". Nutrition in Clinical Practice 25.6 (2010): 634-640. Web. [Accessed 02/01/2016]

Bernhard Watz (2013) Anti-inflammatory Effects of Plant-based Foods and of their Constituents, International Journal for Vitamin and Nutrition Research, Volume 78, pp. 293-298. [Accessed 01/20/2016]

Adam, O et al. (January 2003), Anti-inflammatory effects of a low arachidonic acid diet and fish oil in patients with rheumatoid arthritis, Rheumatology International, Volume 23, Issue 1, pp 27-36 [Accessed 09/03/2016]

www.nutrition.org [Accessed 02/03/2016]

Grzanna, L et al (2005). Ginger—An Herbal Medicinal Product with Broad Anti-Inflammatory Actions, Journal of Medicinal Food. Volume 8, Issue 2: pp. 125-132. [Accessed 01/01/2016]
Arthritis.org. 8 Food Ingredients That Can Cause Inflammation. Available at: http://www.arthritis.org/living-with-arthritis/arthritis-diet/foods-to-avoid-limit/food-ingredients-and-inflammation-12.php [Accessed on 03/29/2016]

NIH (2014) Handout on Health: Rheumatoid Arthritis. Available at: http://www.niams.nih.gov/Health_Info/Rheumatic_Disease/ [Accessed on 04/03/2016]

INDEX

A

Acute Inflammation 8
Allergies 10
Almonds
   Cinema sweet & salty nuts 223
   Fast & fresh granola trail mix 208
   Homemade hot cross buns 222
   Mixed fruit & nut milkshake 95
Apple
   Baked apple & walnut chips 209
   Banana & Apple Blend 84
   Homemade apple tea 92
   Spiced apple & quince sauce 210
   Sweet & savoury smoothie 89
Apricot
   Apricot and coconut wholefood bites 229
   Apricot and Lamb Tagine 115
   Date compote 226
   Fruit pudding 227
Asparagus
   Vegetable Paella 169
Asthma 10
Autoimmune diseases 9
Avocado
   Avocado boat breakfast 38
   Japanese avocado & shrimp salad 182
   On-the-go taco salad 179

B

Banana
   Antioxidant smoothie 86
   Banana & Apple Blend 84
   Grilled banana and nut butter 228
   Sweet & savoury smoothie 89
Beef
   Beef Chili 112
   Chili beef & broccoli beef 108
   Fast & fresh lean beef burgers 103
   Herby chuck roast & scrummy veg 102
   Oriental Beef And Spring Onion Wrap 113
   Siracha Steak Wraps 55
   Slow cooked beef brisket 106
   Thai beef with coconut milk 110
Beetroot
   Brilliantly beetroot flavoured ketchup 202
   Mackerel & beetroot super salad 183, 187
   Roasted beetroot, goats cheese & egg salad 175
Benefits of the diet 13
Black beans
   Cayenne-spiced beans & sweet potato 193
   Latino black bean stew 157
Blueberry
   Antioxidant smoothie 86
   Blueberry and spinach shake 85
   Vanilla and nutmg muffins with blueberries 221
Bok choy
   Bok choy & sesame seed stir fry 166
Broccoli
   Cashew nuts & broccoli snack 200
   Chili beef & broccoli curry 108
   Ginger purple sprouting broccoli 196
   Indian broccoli rabe & cauliflower 165, 173
Brown rice
   Latino black bean stew 157
   Lime & satay tofu with sugersnaps 156
   Portabella mushroom cups 164
   Rustic apricot & walnut rice 206
Brown Rice
   Rainbow Rice Salad 212
Buckwheat 32, 46
   Apricot & Vanilla Pancakes 40
   Brilliant Buckwheat Breakfast 33
Bulgar
   Green Onion & Lemon Bulgar Side Dish 188
Bulgarwheat
   Bulgarwheat, goats cheese & tabbouleh salad 176

C

Cancer 10
Carrot
   Carrots and tart cherry ketchup 198
   Ginger, Carrot & Lime Soup 66
   Spicy cod broth 141
   Sweet & savoury smoothie 89
   Tarragon swede and carrot mash 191
Cashew
   Cashew nuts & broccoli snack 200
Cauliflower
   Indian broccoli rabe & cauliflower 165, 173
   Mustard cauliflower slices 199
Celery
   Super strawberry smoothie 96
   Symptom Soothing Smoothie 87
Cherries
   Fast & fresh granola trail mix 208
   Fruit cocktail with rose water yogurt 225
   Tropical Coconut Delight 30
Chia Seeds
   Chia Berry Superfood 41
   Tropical Coconut Delight 30
   Wonderful watermelon drink 88
Chicken
   Burrito Brunch 59
   Cajun chicken & prawn 118, 130
   Cumin & mango chicken salad 181
   Greek fennel & olive baked chicken 126
   Harissa spiced chicken tray-bake

121
Italian chicken zucchini spaghetti 125
Lebanese chicken kebabs and hummus 124
Marvellous Mini Meatloaves 42
Middle eastern chicken salad 52
Nutty pesto chicken supreme 128
On-the-go taco salad 179
PALEO-FRIENDLY ITALIAN OPEN SANDWICH
   Paleo-Friendly Italian Open Sandwich 60
Rosemary chicken & sweet potato stew 127
Super sesame chicken noodles 123
Tomato & olive chicken fiesta 117
Winter warming chunky chicken soup 72

Chickpeas
   Bulgarwheat, goats cheese & tabbouleh salad 176
   Homemade moroccan hummus 190
   Lebanese chicken kebabs and hummus 124

Chilli
   Ginger & chili sea bass fillets 134

Coconut
   Apricot and coconut wholefood bites 229

Coconut Milk
   Coconut, banana and raspberry hot milk 230
   Tropical Coconut Delight 30

Cod
   Spicy Cod Broth 141
   Tasty Thai Broth 69

Couscous
   Curried Couscous 214

Cranberries
   Spinach, orange & cranberry salad 177

Cranberry
   Fresh cranberry & lime juice 93
   Watercress, Orange And Cranberry Salad 217

Cucumber
   Antioxidant smoothie 86
   Symptom soothing smoothie 87

Cumin
   Toasted cumin crunch 159
   Curried Chickpeas & Yogurt Dip 54

D

Dates
   Date compote COMPOTE 226
   Fruit & nut slices 233
   Pecan & date snack bars 236

Diabetes 9

Duck
   Chinese orange-spiced duck breasts 120

E

Egg
   Coconut Pancakes 242
   Spiced Pumpkin Pancakes 215

Eggs
   Gluten-Free Vanilla Crepes 36
   Make your own pizza 104
   Mediterranean Vegetable Frittata 37
   Oriental Cabbage & Egg Roll 58
   Protein Scotch Eggs 44
   Sweetcorn & mushroom frittata 43

F

Farro
   Farro & tomato pilaf 205

fennel
   Fresh tuna steak & fennel salad 143
   Greek fennel & olive baked chicken 126

Foods to avoid or cut down 16
Foods to buy 18

G

Ginger
   Blackberry & ginger milkshake 90
   Ginger, Carrot & Lime Soup 66
   Ginger & chili sea bass fillets 134

Goats cheese
   Bulgarwheat, goats cheese & tabbouleh salad 176
   Roasted beetroot, goats cheese & egg salad 175

Granola
   Fast & fresh granola trail mix 208

Grapes
   Mutli-vitamin smoothie 83, 98

Greek Yogurt
   Citrus yogurt bircher 39

H

Haddock
   Smoked haddock & pea risotto 135

Halibut 142
   Baked garlic & lemon halibut 142

Heart Disease 10

I

Inflammation 7
   Chronic Inflammation 8

K

Kale
   Flaversome Vegetarian Tagine 71
   Spinach & kale breaded balls 197
   Super strawberry smoothie 96

Kidney beans
   Rustic garlic and chive quinoa 163

Kipper
   Kipper & celery salad 178

L

Lamb
   Apricot and Lamb Tagine 115
   Lovely lamb burgers & minty yogurt 105
   Lush lamb & rosemary casserole 111
   Super lamb shoulder with apricot & zucchini mash 107
Langoustine
   Spanish Langoustine Paella 57
Lentils
   Curried lentil & spinach stew 73
   Moroccan spiced lentil soup 70
Lime
   Ginger, Carrot & Lime Soup 66

M

Mackerel
   Mackerel & beetroot super salad 183, 187
Mahi-Mahi
   Sesame Mahi-Mahi & Fruit Salsa 144
Mango
   Cumin & mango chicken salad 181
Mint
   Mutli-vitamin smoothie 83, 98
Mushrooms
   Asian Squash & Shittake Soup 67
   Portabella mushroom cups 164
Mutiple Sclerosis 9

O

Obesity 10
Olive
   Tomato & olive chicken fiesta 117
Oranges
   Spiced oranges 224

P

Pasta
   Sun dried tomato & nut pasta 161
Pea
   Smoked haddock & pea risotto 135
Peaches
   Blackberry & ginger milkshake 90
   Mutli-vitamin smoothie 83, 98
   Spiced Peaches 241
Pecans
   Pecan & date snack bars 236
Peppers
   Spiced red pepper & tomato soup 68
Pineapple
   Fresh tropical juice 94
   Symptom soothing smoothie 87
Pinenuts
   Lemony taro dip 204
Pork
   Mighty herb pork meatballs 109
Prawn
   Cajun chicken & prawn 118, 130
Prunes
   Fruit pudding 227
Pumpkin
   Spiced pumpkin pancakes 231
   Spiced Pumpkin Pancakes 215
Pumpkin seeds
   Roasted paprika pumpkin seeds 207

Q

Quinoa
   Burrito Brunch 59
   Latino black bean stew 157
   Mexican spice infused quinoa 194, 213
   Nutmeg & Cherry Breakfast Quinoa 34
   Rustic garlic and chive quinoa 163

R

Rheumatoid Arthritis 9
Rice
   Farro & tomato pilaf 205

S

Salmon
   Salmon & Lime with Arugula 140
   Sizzling salmon & green salad 180
   Smoked salmon hash browns 145
   Wasabi salmon burger 139
Salsa
   Mexican Salsa 216
Sardines
   Citrus & herb sardines 148, 153
Scallops 146, 152
   Scrumptious scallops with cilantro and lime 146, 152
Sea Bass
   Ginger & chili sea bass fillets 134
Sesame seed
   Bok choy & sesame seed stir fry 166
Shark
   Spicy shark steaks 149
Shimp
   Gluten-free coconut shrimp bites 147
   Japanese avocado & shrimp salad 182
   Parsley & lemon spanish shrimp 137
   Shrimp & Zucchini Noodle Jars 56

Soy Milk
 Warming Gingerbread Oatmeal 31
Spaghetti squash
 Spaghetti squash & marinated tempah 162
Spinach
 Blueberry and spinach shake 85
 Curried lentil & spinach stew 73
 Nutty pesto chicken supreme 128
 Spinach & kale breaded balls 197
 Spinach, orange and cranberry salad 177
 Super tofu & spinach scramble 185
Squash
 North African Spaghetti Squash 170
Stock
 Homemade Vegetable Stock 76
Strawberries
 Fruit cocktail with rose water yogurt 225
 Lemon lavender & strawberry compote 235
 Mixed fruit & nut milkshake 95
 Strawberry and banana pudding 220
Swede
 Tarragon swede and carrot mash 191
Sweet Potato
 Cayenne-spiced beans & sweet potato 193
 Flaversome vegetarian tagine 71
 Mackerel & beetroot super salad 183, 187
 Mediterranean Vegetable Frittata 37
 Mustard & tarragon sweet potato salad 186
 Rosemary chicken & sweet potato stew 127
 Smoked salmon hash browns 145
 Super healthy sweet potato fries 192

T

Tapioca starch
 Make your own pizza 104
Taro
 Lemony taro dip 204
Tempah
 Spaghetti squash & marinated tempah 162
 Spicy vegetable burgers 160
Tilapia
 Nut-crust tilapia with kale 138
Tofu
 Lime & satay tofu with sugersnaps 156
 Super tofu & spinach scramble 185
 Zucchini & pepper lasagna 158
Tomatoes
 Spiced red pepper & tomato soup 68
 Sun dried tomato & nut pasta 161
Tuna Steak
 Fresh tuna steak & fennel salad 143
Turkey
 Healthy turkey gumbo 119
 Marvellous Mini Meatloaves 42
 Protein Scotch Eggs 44
 Terrific turkey burgers 122
Turnip
 Tasty turnip chips 195

W

Walnut
 Apricot and coconut wholefood bites 229
 Baked apple & walnut chips 209
 Walnut & dark chocolate chip cookies 219
Wasabi
 Wasabi salmon burger 139
Watermelon
 Wonderful watermelon drink 88
Wholemeal oats
 Brilliant Buckwheat Breakfast 33
 Citrus yogurt bircher 39
 Peanut cereal bars 232
 Tropical Coconut Delight 30
 Warming Gingerbread Oatmeal 31

Z

Zucchini
 Italian chicken & zucchini spaghetti 125
 Mediterranean Vegetable Frittata 37
 Shrimp & Zucchini Noodle Jars 56
 Super lamb shoulder with apricot & zucchini mash 107
 Vegetable Paella 169
 Zainy zucchini ketchup 203
 Zucchini & pepper lasagna 158

www.ingramcontent.com/pod-product-compliance
Lightning Source LLC
Chambersburg PA
CBHW080322170426
43193CB00017B/2877